Thieme

Atlas of Middle Ear Surgery

Michel Gersdorff, MD, PhD
Professor and Director
Department of Otolaryngology
St. Luc University Hospital
Brussels, Belgium

Jean-Marc Gérard, MD
Attending Otoneurosurgeon
Department of Otolaryngology
St. Luc University Hospital
Brussels, Belgium

254 illustrations

Thieme
Stuttgart · New York

Important note: Medicine is an ever-changing science undergoing continual development. Research and clinical experience are continually expanding our knowledge, in particular our knowledge of proper treatment and drug therapy. Insofar as this book mentions any dosage or application, readers may rest assured that the authors, editors, and publishers have made every effort to ensure that such references are in accordance with **the state of knowledge at the time of production of the book**. Nevertheless, this does not involve, imply, or express any guarantee or responsibility on the part of the publishers in respect to any dosage instructions and forms of applications stated in the book. **Every user is requested to examine carefully** the manufacturers' leaflets accompanying each drug and to check, if necessary in consultation with a physician or specialist, whether the dosage schedules mentioned therein or the contraindications stated by the manufacturers differ from the statements made in the present book. Such examination is particularly important with drugs that are either rarely used or have been newly released on the market. Every dosage schedule or every form of application used is entirely at the user's own risk and responsibility. The authors and publishers request every user to report to the publishers any discrepancies or inaccuracies noticed. If errors in this work are found after publication, errata will be posted at www.thieme.com on the product description page.

Library of Congress Cataloging-in-Publication Data
is available from the publisher.

Illustrator: Anne Johnson, M.S.M.I. (Master of Science in Medical Illustration), WAG Design & Communications, Lasne, Belgium

Rüdigerstrasse 14, 70469 Stuttgart, Germany
http://www.thieme.de
Thieme New York, 333 Seventh Avenue,
New York, NY 10001, USA
http://www.thieme.com

Cover design: Thieme Publishing Group
Typesetting by primustype Hurler, Notzingen, Germany
Printed in India by Gopsons Paper Ltd., Delhi
ISBN 978-3-13-145041-8

1 2 3 4 5 6

Foreword 1

It is a privilege for me to write a foreword for this excellent book, *Atlas of Middle Ear Surgery.*

This book is written for the otorhinolaryngologist. It is arranged in seven sections and very well illustrated so that the reader can sequentially follow the pathophysiology and surgical management of the various pathological entities that affect the middle ear. It contains specific details regarding each disease, which makes this atlas also useful as a reference.

Continuing improvements in our ability to treat disorders of the middle ear are based on the constant advances in science. These innovations have made it possible for us to bring more and more relief to our patients and this book beautifully portrays these advances and fills a real need in the area of continuous education in our specialty.

Through the leadership of Professor Michel Gersdorff, an expert clinician and surgeon, this work presents the current art and science of surgical treatment of middle ear disorders, including the different and sometimes controversial surgical treatments and their complications.

Antonio De la Cruz, MD † (1944–2009)
Former Director of Education House Ear Institute
Former Professor of Clinical Otolaryngology, University of Southern California
President, American Otological Society 2007
Président International, Institut George Portmann, Bordeaux, France 2002-2005
President, American Academy of Otolaryngology Head and Neck Surgery, 1998

Authors' note: Our book was already in production when we learned of the death of our esteemed colleague and friend, Dr Antonio de la Cruz, renowned international otologist of exceptional charisma. He very kindly wrote this short introduction, which we are of course including in this book. We are happy to have had the opportunity to thank him in person.

Foreword 2

It is a great honor and privilege to have been invited by Professor Michel Gersdorff and Jean-Marc Gérard to write a foreword to this atlas on middle ear surgery.

As head of a medical school as prestigious as St. Luc University Hospital, Professor Gersdorff's writing of this book marks the culmination of a long and distinguished career and demonstrates:

- His willingness to synthesize his consummate knowledge and bring it to fruition;
- His desire to communicate this knowledge and experience to a larger audience.

This book is a model of balance, rigor, and elegance:

- Balance and harmony between the text and illustrations that make it easy to read, yet highly educational
- Rigor in the choice of words and selection of operative procedures which allow reproducible results
- Elegance in the esthetic quality of its iconography and page layout

I would like to thank Professor Gersdorff for accomplishing this ambitious project for the benefit of the entire otorhinolaryngological community and, more particularly, young otological surgeons seeking a book of reference.

Bernard Fraysse, MD, PhD
Director, Department of Otorhinolaryngology,
University Hospital Purpan,
Toulouse, France

Preface 1

Having spent many years at the University of Louvain teaching otology to medical students, future otorhinolaryngologists, and visiting doctors, it seems only natural that I should write a book about middle ear surgery, the most frequently performed surgery by ENT specialists.

The surgical techniques described here are those performed in our teaching hospital on a routine basis. Some are original, while others are the fruits of training with my mentors and colleagues during professional sojourns, congresses, and meetings.

As with any craft, the craftsman's skill is a direct reflection of the diversity of his education and experience, as well as a tribute to his unwavering dedication. My mentor in otology, to whom I remain eternally grateful, was Professor Michel Portmann of Bordeaux. He taught me not only the philosophy and clinical techniques involved, but also the importance of audacity, the value of listening, and the meaning of friendship.

In the early days of my career, I drew upon the knowledge and mastery of numerous talented surgeons, many of whom made a deep and lasting impression on me. They include, in order of acquaintance, Jean-Marie Sterkers, Claude Henri Chouard, Guy Lacher, Bill House, Howard House, Jim Sheehy, Jean Marquet, Ugo Fish, and Christian Deguine, to name a few.

Later, many others from my own generation both inspired and enriched my work. They have since become good friends of mine in the tight-knit world of international otology. I will not mention them by name, but they know who they are.

I sincerely hope this small book on middle ear surgery will be of use to young otological surgeons seeking to avail themselves of the know-how and expertise of their more experienced counterparts. While it may not be perfect, this book is nevertheless honest and direct, describing concrete and validated surgical techniques. Do not expect to find descriptions of rarely used procedures yielding hypothetical and random results. I trust the tips provided will prove helpful.

My thanks go to Jean-Marc Gérard, my colleague and collaborator. I greatly appreciate the quality of his work and wish him every success in his promising career. Thanks also to Anne Johnson, our talented illustrator, who worked tirelessly on this project, and our publisher Thieme, who believed in us from the start.

Happy reading!

Michel Gersdorff, MD, PhD

Preface 2

I would like to thank my mentor, Professor Michel Gersdorff, for giving me the opportunity to be his pupil and collaborator. He is indeed a great teacher and a true gentleman. I would also like to thank Gilbert Chantrain, Marie-Paule Thill, and my father, Michel Gérard, all of them ENT surgeons, for introducing me to this discipline and conveying to me their passion for their craft. Special thanks too to my wife, Rachel, and two daughters, Lola and Freya, for being so understanding about the long hours my work entails. Finally, I hope readers will appreciate the beautiful illustrations so skillfully executed by my friend Anne Johnson.

Jean-Marc Gérard, MD

Table of Contents

1

Anatomy and Physiopathology of the Middle Ear

1__Anatomy and Physiopathology of the Middle Ear

Practical and Surgical Anatomy

Retroauricular View

Fig. 1.1

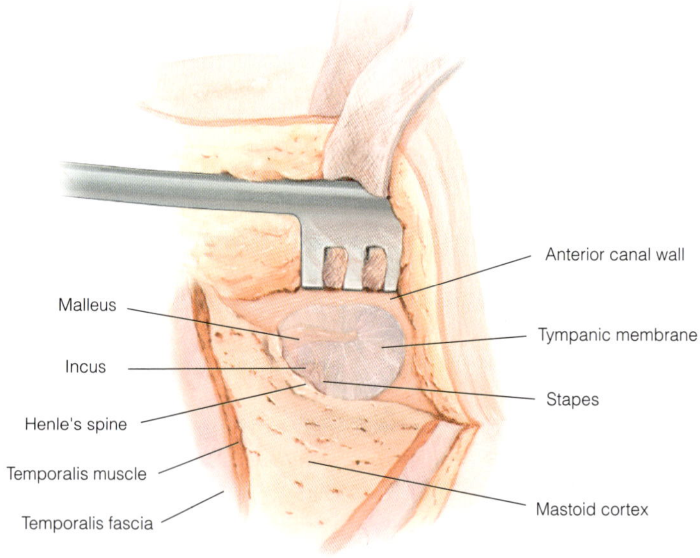

Fig. 1.1

Transmeatal View

Fig. 1.2

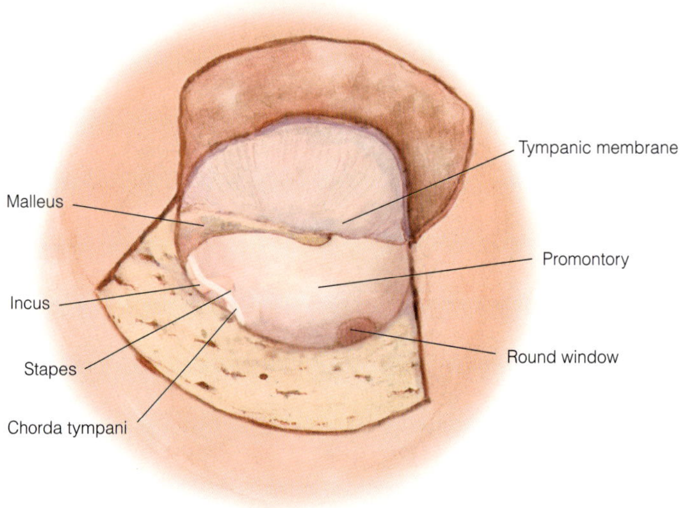

Fig. 1.2

Stapes Surgery View

Fig. 1.3

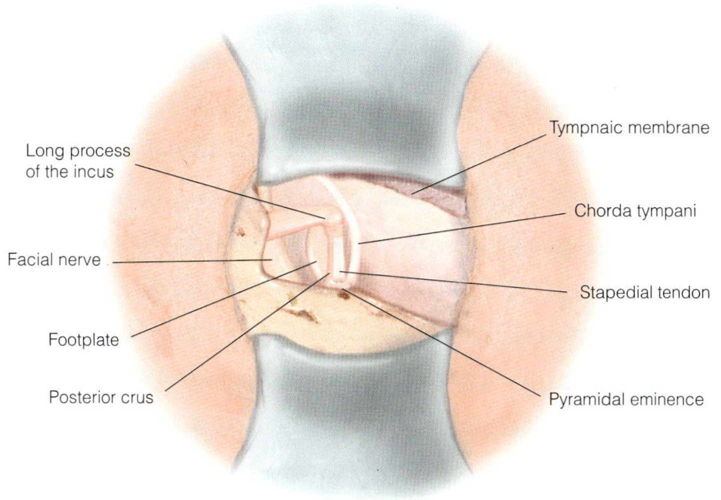

Fig. 1.3

Transmastoid View

Fig. 1.4

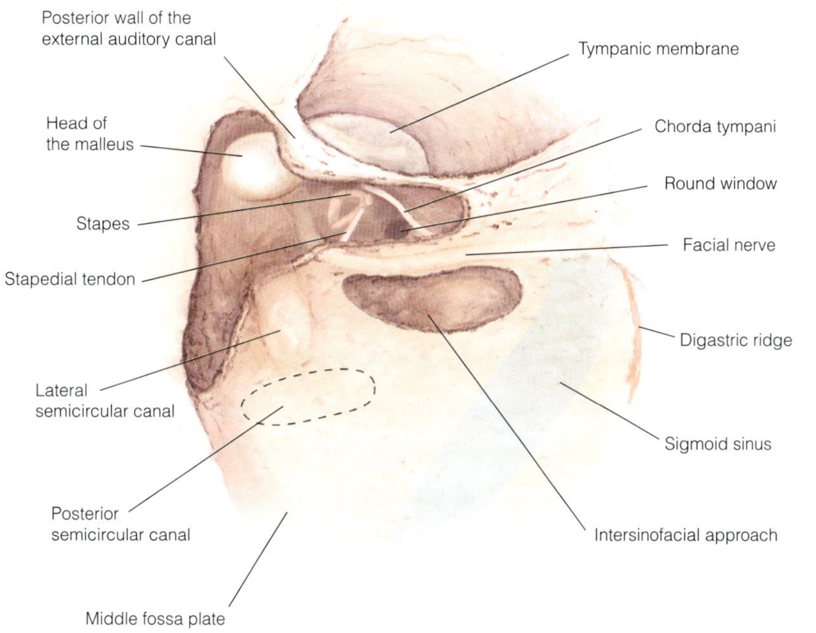

Fig. 1.4

Canal-Wall-Down View

Fig. 1.5

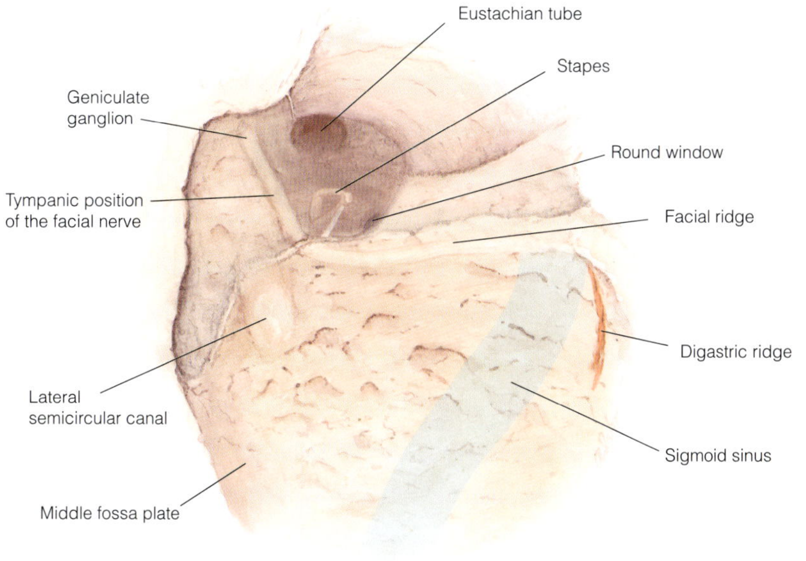

Fig. 1.5

Physiopathology

Definition of Chronic Otitis Media

Chronic otitis media is an inflammatory condition of the middle ear cavities which lasts for more than 3 months and generates morphological sequelae.

The term chronic otitis media includes:

- Chronic otitis media with effusion
- Active chronic otitis media (suppurative)
- Dry tympanic membrane perforation with or without ossicular chain problems
- Tympanosclerosis
- Atelectasis (retraction pockets)
- Cholesteatomatous chronic otitis media

Pathogenesis of Chronic Otitis Media

This inflammatory process starts in the middle ear mucosa and given a favorable environment, such as mesenchymal and gas exchange alterations, develops into a chronic clinical entity. Mesenchymal and gas exchange alterations result from various processes.

The first process is embryological. When resorption and/or condensation of the mesenchyma are disturbed, this leads to developmental disorders of the middle ear cavity, such as mastoid pneumatization and inappropriate drainage of residual mucus. Alteration of the mesenchyma's role as a carrier and support for epidermal migration results in poor quality of the lamina propria, weakening the tympanic membrane.

Anatomically, attic regions are separated by bony–membranous barriers, which allow ventilation of their various compartments.

Small openings interfere with their ventilation.

Histologically, the middle ear is divided into an anteroinferior compartment, the cell function of which mainly focuses on mucociliary clearance, and a posteroinferior compartment, with cells involved in gas exchange. When inflammation occurs, these two functions are disturbed, leading to increased mucus and viscosity as well as pressure imbalance (negative pressure). The resulting mucosal inflammation, arising directly from bacterial infection or indirectly from viral infection, increases the chronic inflammatory environment of chronic otitis media.

Middle Ear Ventilation

The different ventilation pathways of the middle ear cavities are illustrated in Figs. 1.6 to 1.9. Anatomical or acquired dysfunction of these ventilation pathways can explain the different types and evolutions of cholesteatoma (see Classifications, p. 106).

Figs. 1.6–1.9

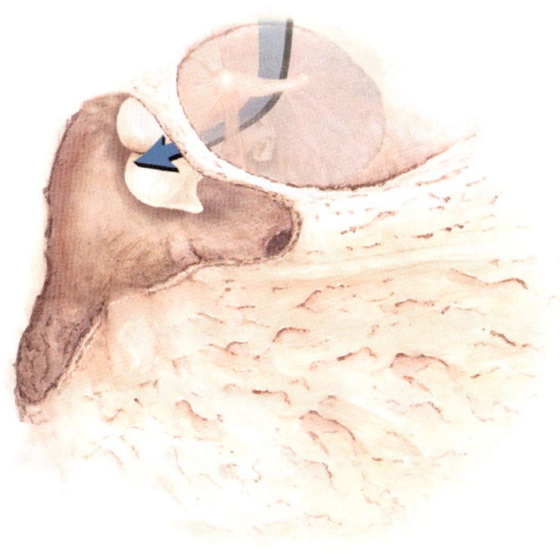

Fig. 1.6

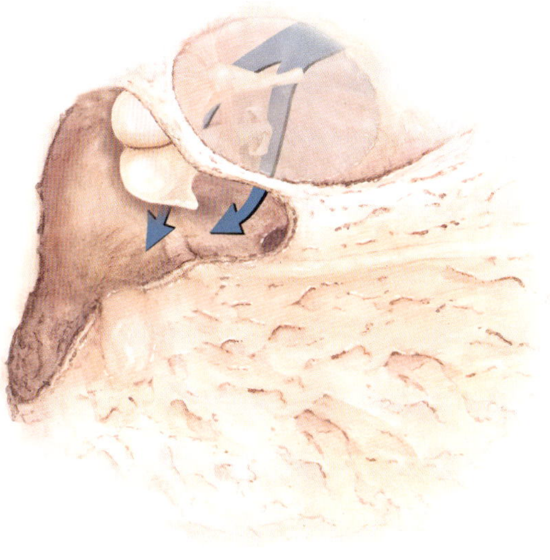

Fig. 1.7

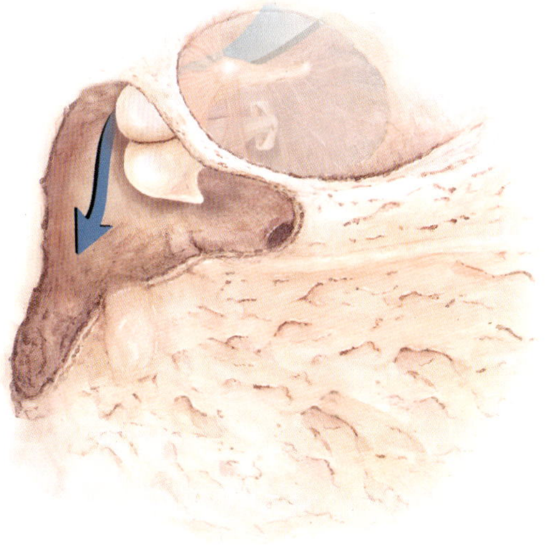

Fig. 1.8

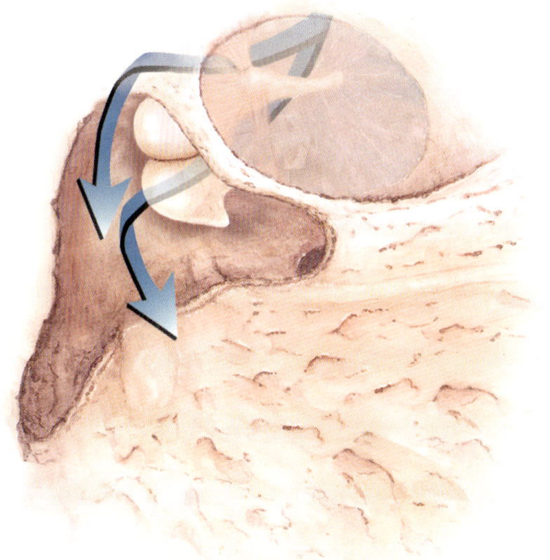

Fig. 1.9

Physiopathogenesis of Cholesteatoma

A cholesteatoma is a mass of keratin (skin) in the middle ear cavities which consists of a perimatrix and a matrix. There are at least three kinds of cholesteatoma in the middle ear, resulting from invagination (retraction pocket), migration, or congenital inclusion. A cholesteatoma goes through three successive inflammatory phases, the first resulting in a retraction pocket, the second leading to pathology of the epidermis and lower external auditory canal, and the third—the actual cholesteatoma—involving invasion and autodestruction (bone lysis) of the middle ear. In this last phase, many factors play a role: collagenosis, osteoclasts, cytokines, nitric oxide, bacteria and their biofilms, and rupture of the retraction pocket. In summary, cholesteatoma is an inflammatory disorder of the middle ear characterized by bone resorption.

2

Anesthesia and Surgical Field

2__Anesthesia and Surgical Field

General Anesthesia

The choice of anesthesia depends on the patient, the pathology, the type of surgery, and the surgeon's and anesthetist's usual practice and their experience.

In the majority of cases, general anesthesia is used. Local anesthesia is employed in simple cases, such as transcanal functional revision surgery or transcanal myringoplasty in adults.

General anesthesia is always combined with infiltration of local anesthetic.

Local Anesthesia

Injection Technique

Local anesthesia is achieved by injection of 1% lidocaine and epinephrine 5 µg/mL prior to sterilization and draping.

The Plester technique is used (Plester 1963), which consists of four subperiosteal injections to the ear canal wall at 12, 3, 6, and 9 o'clock.

Fig. 2.1

If a retroauricular approach is taken, the retroauricular fold and mastoid region are injected subcutaneously.

Harvesting of conchal or tragal cartilage requires infiltration of the posterior surface of the auricle or the tragal region.

Tip: Take care not to inject too much into the meatus at 6 o'clock, and palpate the mastoid tip so as not to inject anteroinferiorly, causing facial nerve block.

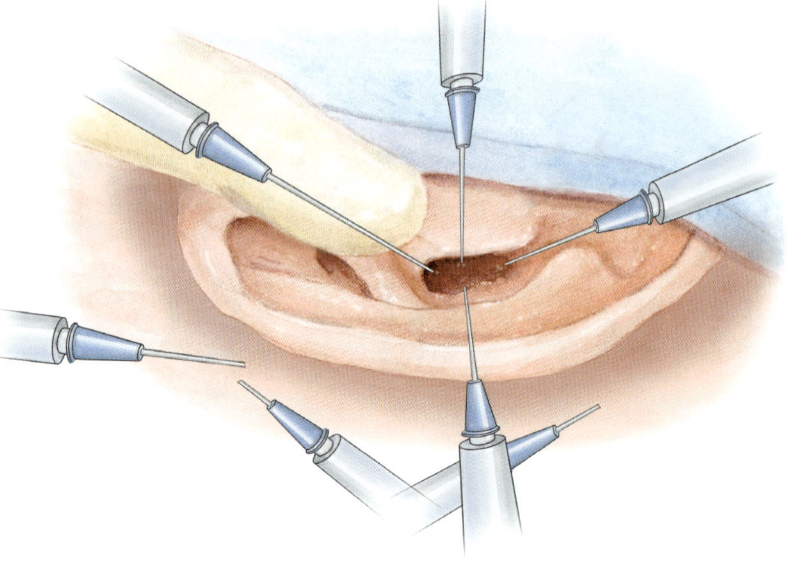

Fig. 2.1

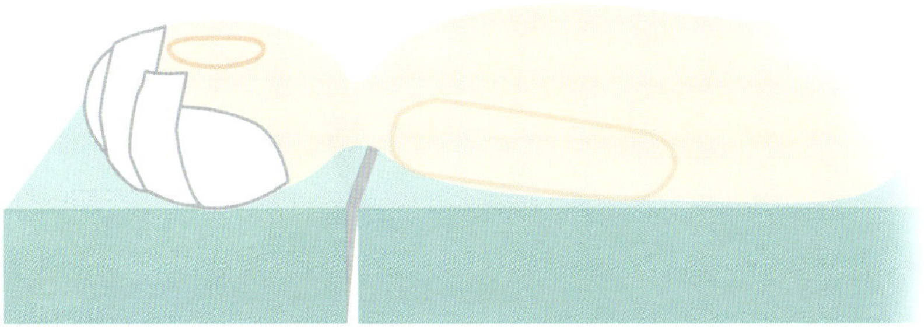

Fig. 2.2

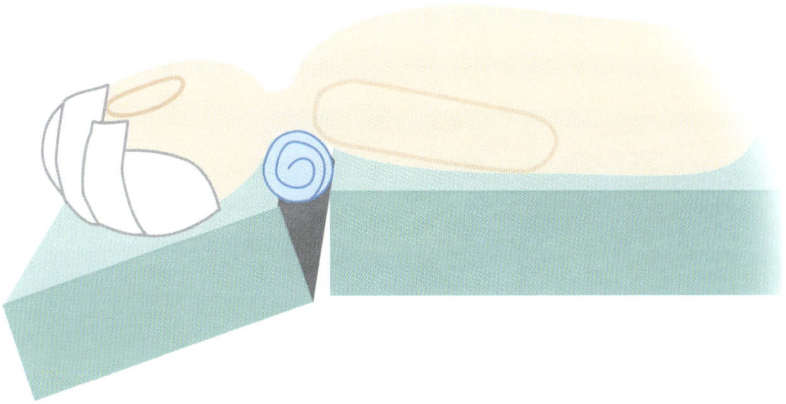

Fig. 2.3

Surgical Field

Tympanoplasty, Head Position

In tympanoplasty, the head position requires a horizontal mastoid presentation.

Fig. 2.2

Stapes Surgery, Head Position

In stapes surgery, the head must be in hyperextension to allow the surgeon a better view of the stapes region. Contralateral rotation of the head to the side must be 45° without interfering with venous circulation.

Fig. 2.3

For the retroauricular approach, the patient's hair is shaved up to 2 cm from the auricular fold. Adhesive tape delimits the surgical field, secures the hair, and facilitates adhesion of the surgical drapes.

Tip: If the patient's neck is stiff, the head rotation can be held by fixing a tape transversely across the forehead. The shoulder is pushed down as far as possible. The patient should be positioned in a few degrees anti-Trendelenburg (10° to 20°) to improve venous circulation.

Operating Room

Room Layout

The microscope is positioned at the head of the operating table, with the scrub nurse and instrument table opposite the surgeon. The motor, laser, and monitoring device are placed alongside the patient's legs, together with the anesthetic equipment.

Fig. 2.4

Tip: During surgery, only the table is moved. Do not turn the patient's head.

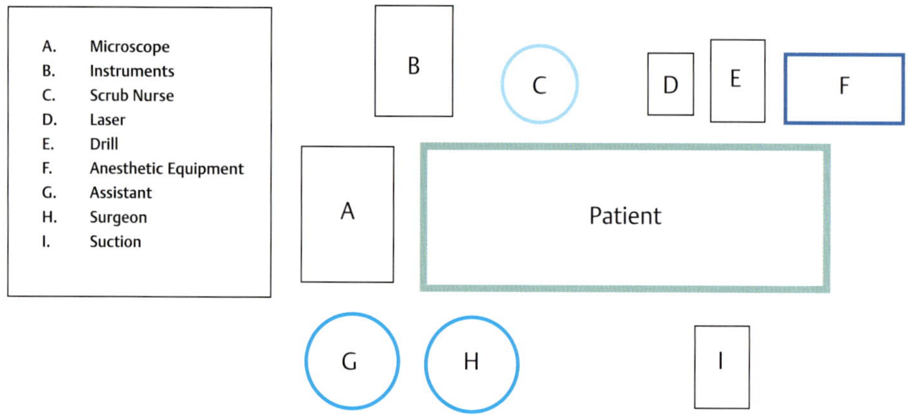

Fig. 2.4

The operating table should be able to rotate forward and backward and move up and down (Trendelenburg and anti-Trendelenburg positions), depending on the surgeon's position.

The surgeon's forearms should be parallel to the floor and supported by the patient's shoulders and table or arm rests, with his or her hands on the patient's head.

3

Surgical Materials

3__Surgical Materials

Surgical Tools

Microscope

Tip: Balance the microscope so it can be moved with the nose and ensure the lenses are well adjusted and clean.

Our microscope is equipped with lateral binocular eyepieces on one side and a video camera connected to a computer with recording software and a CD and DVD burner on the other.

We use a 250-mm lens, except in stapes surgery where a 200-mm lens is preferred. The microscope is draped with a sterile plastic cover.

Instruments

Tip: The scrub nurse should be sufficiently trained to allow the surgeon to remain focused on the microscope at all times.

We use straight instruments, except sometimes to work on the stapes or footplate, where angled ones are more suitable. Lempert suction tubes are used for drilling, except for precision work. Microsuction is used for the middle ear cavity and precise mastoid surgery. Single-use microsuctions with a diameter less than 0.7 mm are used around fragile and precarious structures, such as the footplate, stapes, round window, and in labyrinthine fistula. Low-volume irrigation is performed with a 20-mL syringe and important irrigation with a continuous-flow perfusion. Monopolar coagulation is used for macroscopic work, and a microcoagulation needle at a low power setting for microscopic work. Figs. 3.1–3.29

Basic Instruments

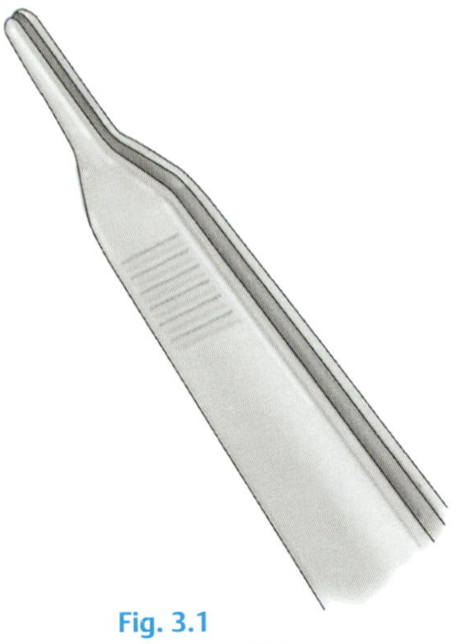

Fig. 3.1
Anatomical forceps

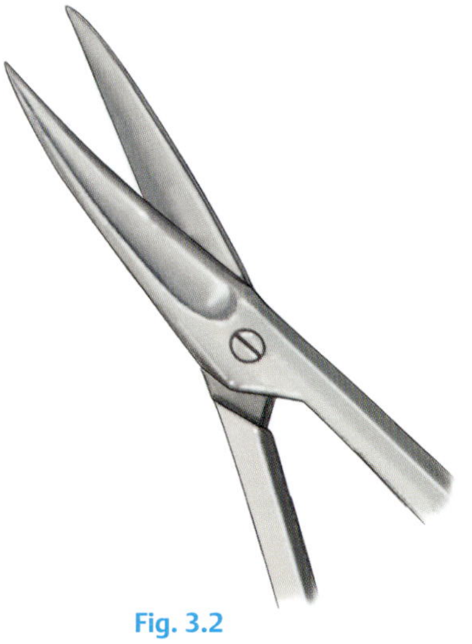

Fig. 3.2
Blunt curved scissors

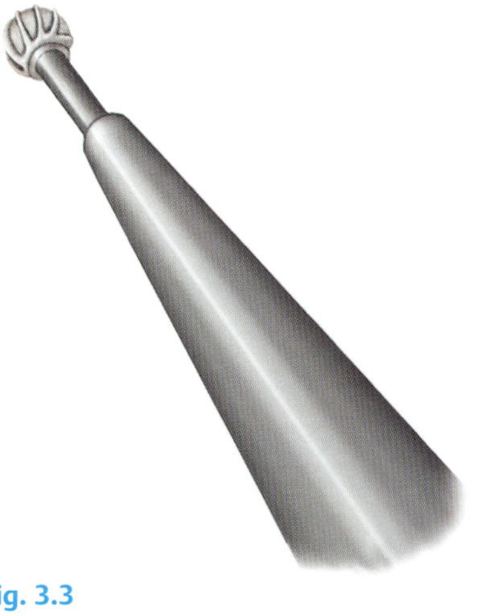

Fig. 3.3
Cutting burr

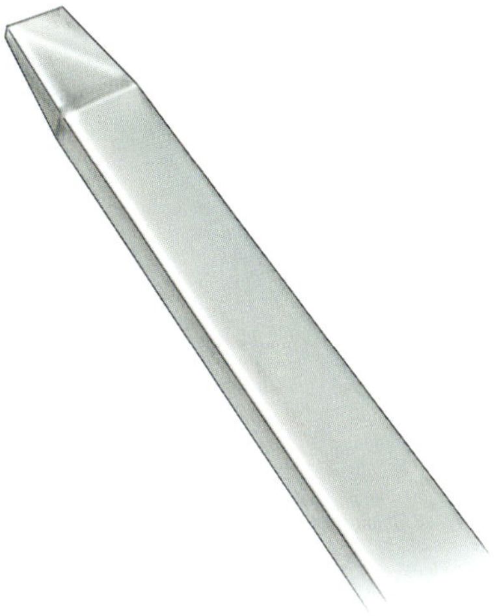

Fig. 3.4
Chisel

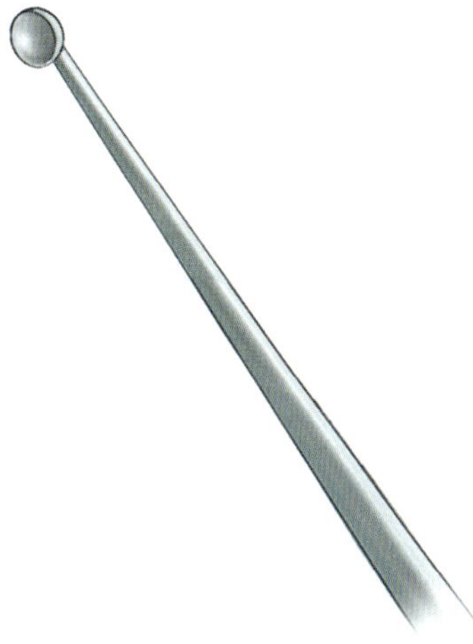

Fig. 3.5
Curette

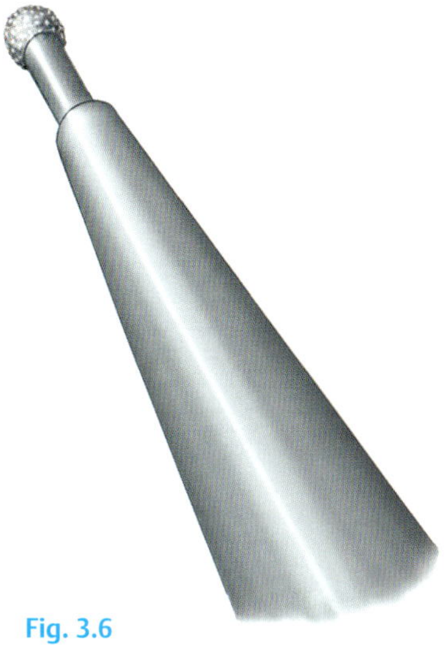

Fig. 3.6
Diamond burr

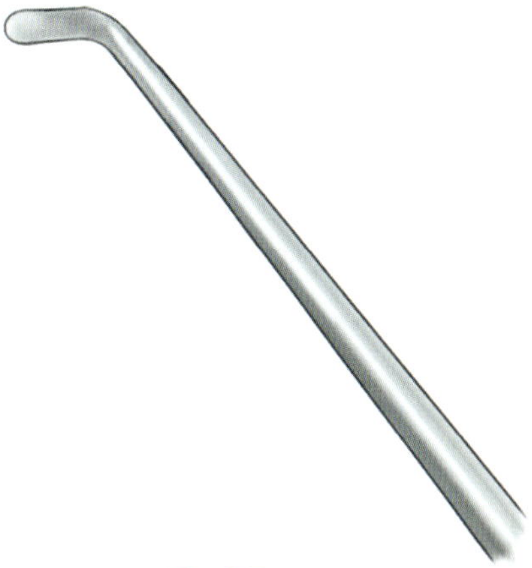

Fig. 3.7
Dissector-elevator

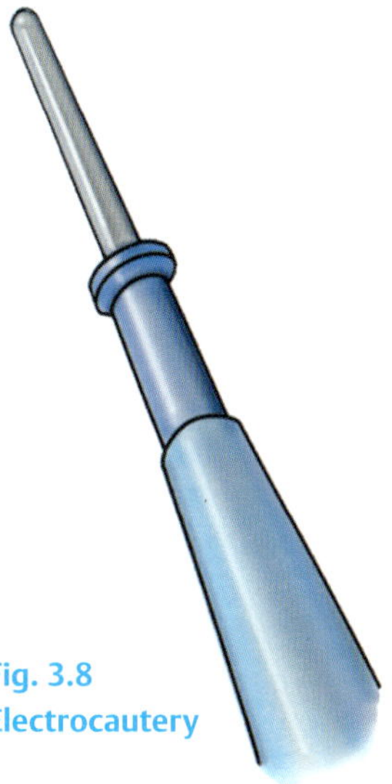

Fig. 3.8
Electrocautery

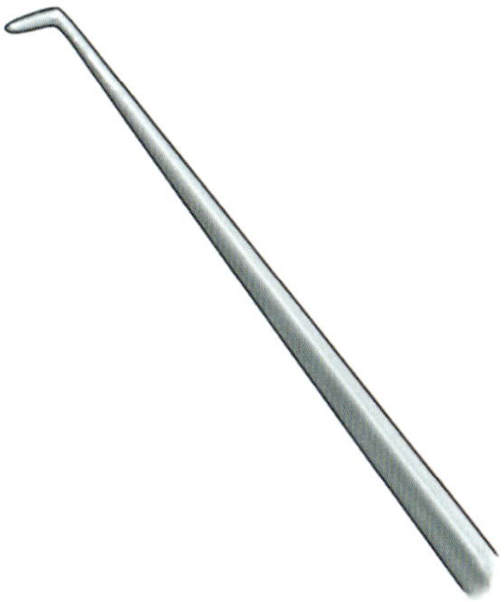

Fig. 3.9
Electrocautery needle

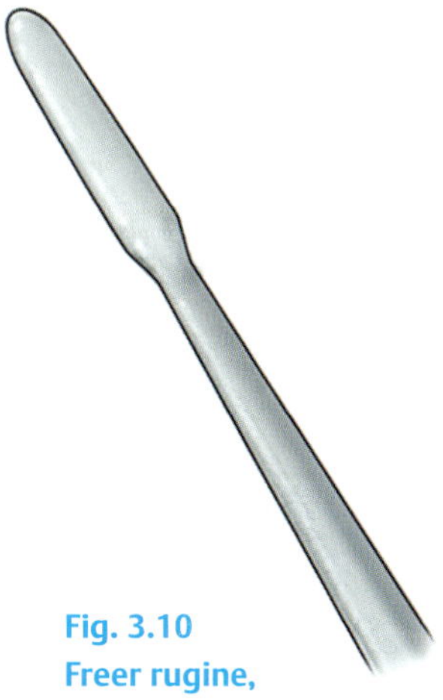

Fig. 3.10
Freer rugine,
periosteal elevator,
raspatory.

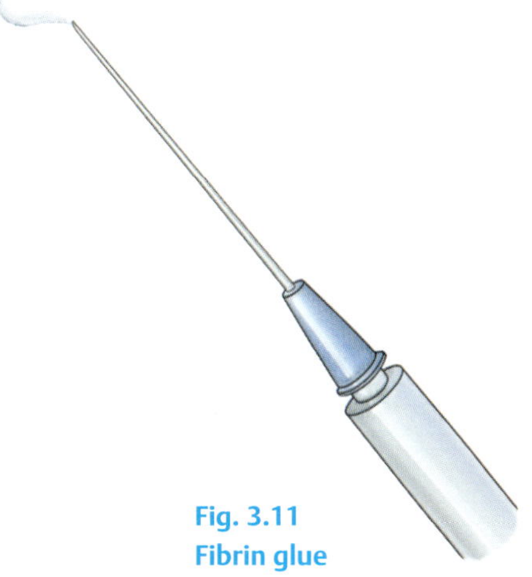

Fig. 3.11
Fibrin glue

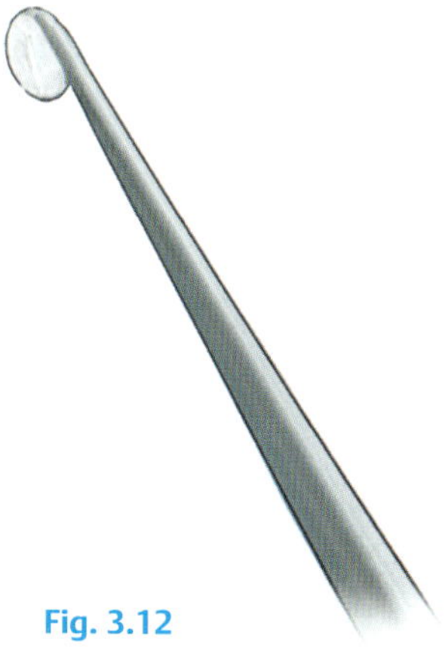

Fig. 3.12
Lateral knife

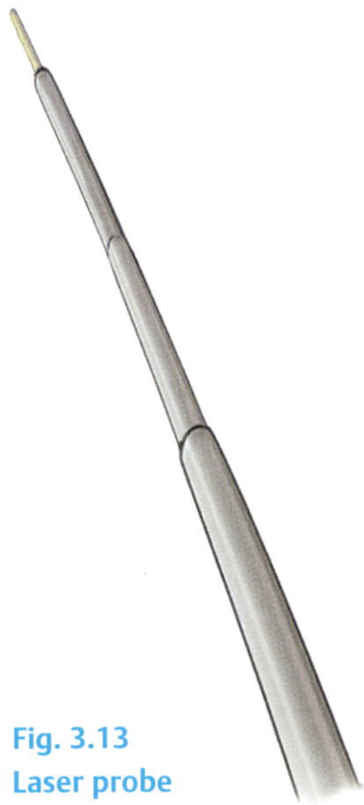

Fig. 3.13
Laser probe

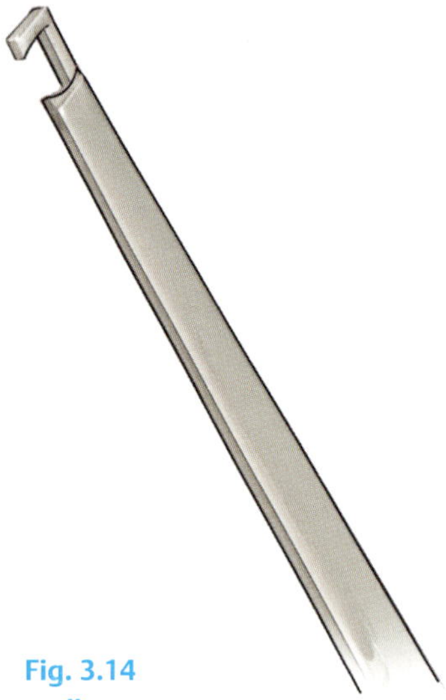

Fig. 3.14
Malleus nipper

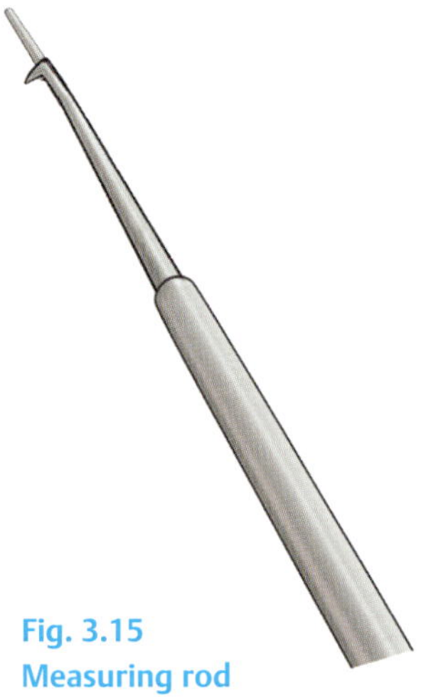

Fig. 3.15
Measuring rod

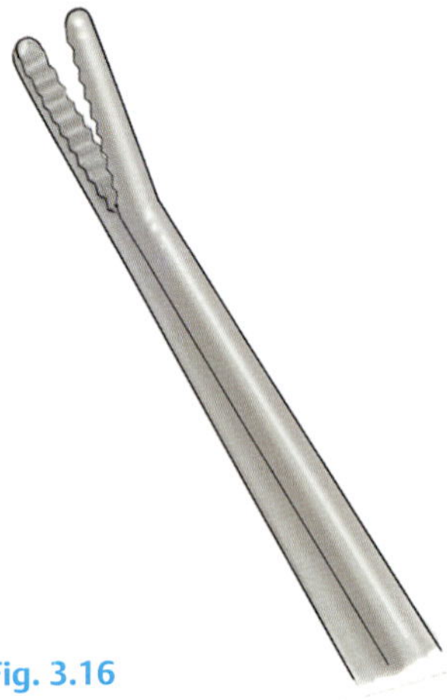

Fig. 3.16
Microforceps

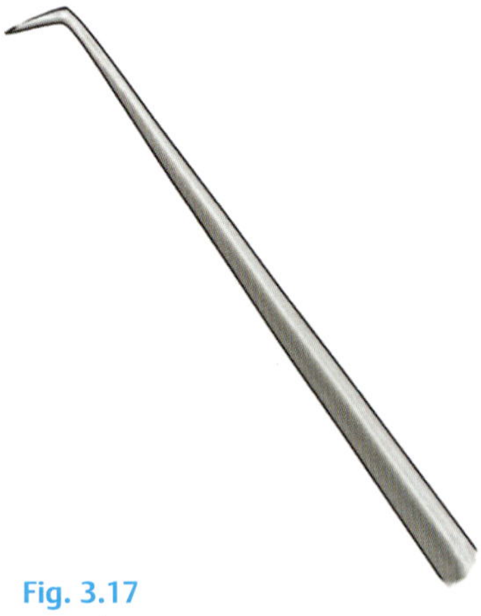

Fig. 3.17
Microhook or small hook

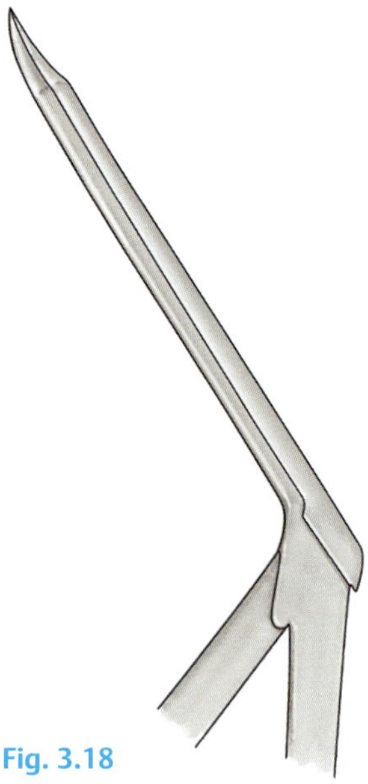

Fig. 3.18
Microscissors

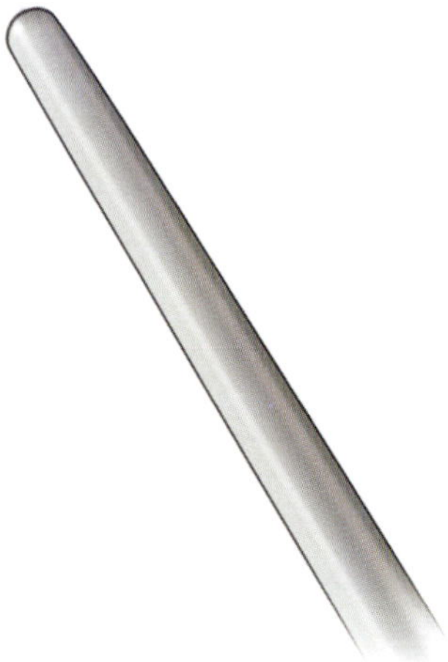

Fig. 3.19
Microsuction

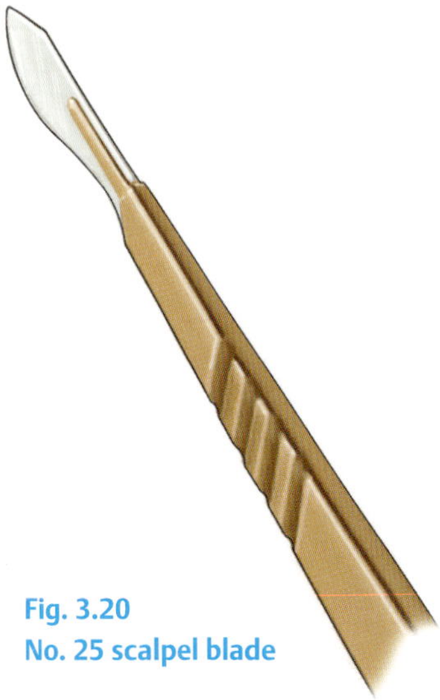

Fig. 3.20
No. 25 scalpel blade

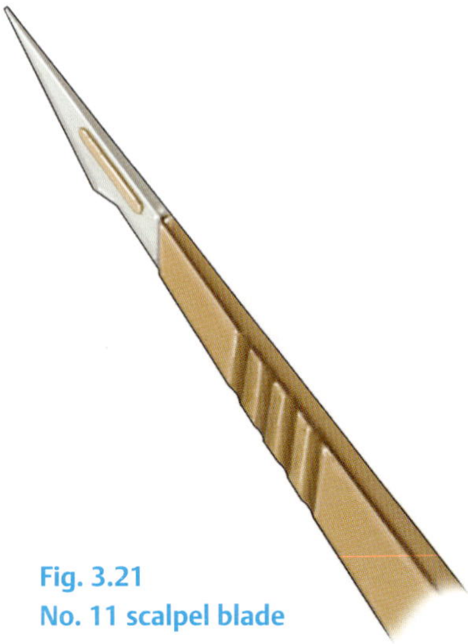

Fig. 3.21
No. 11 scalpel blade

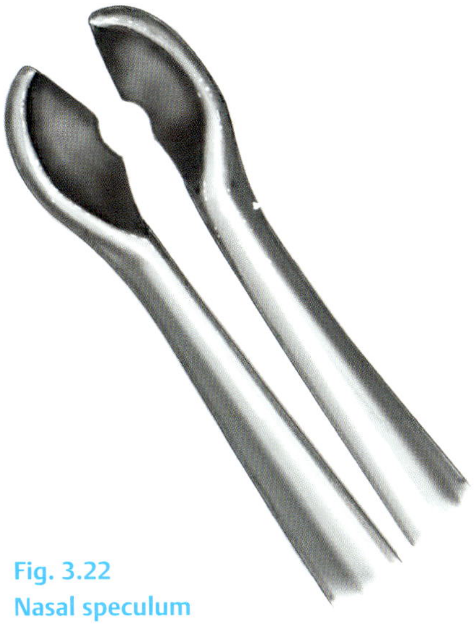

Fig. 3.22
Nasal speculum

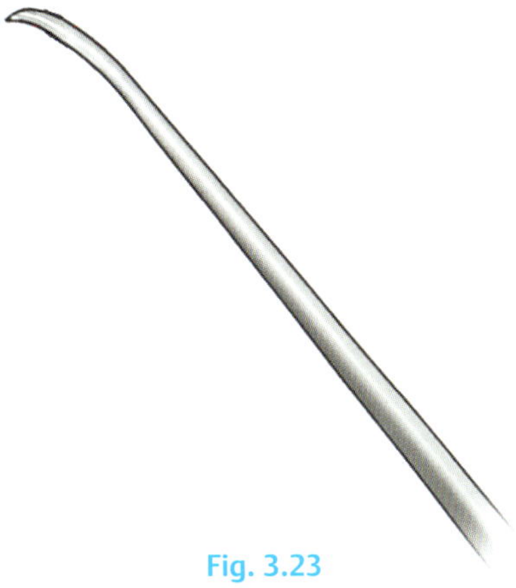

Fig. 3.23
Needle

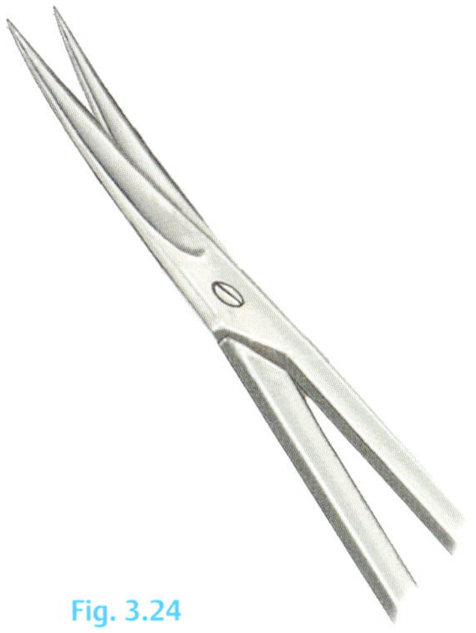

Fig. 3.24
Pointed curved scissors

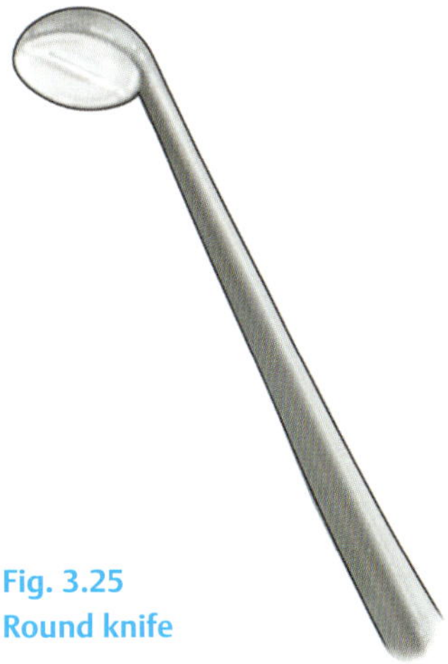

Fig. 3.25
Round knife

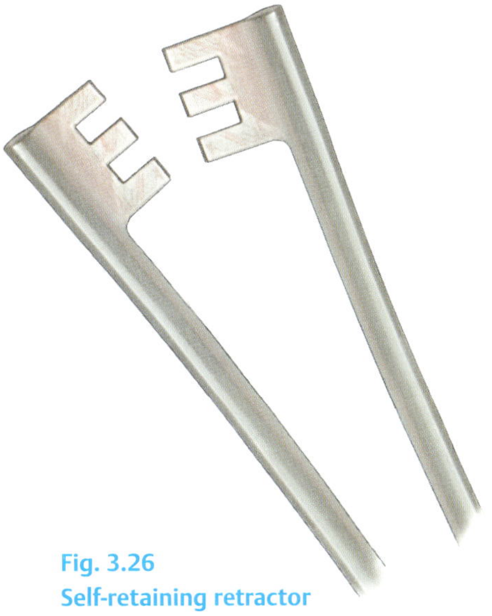

Fig. 3.26
Self-retaining retractor

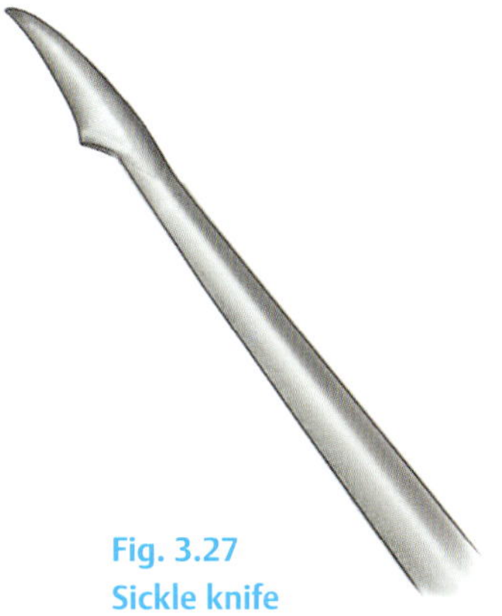

Fig. 3.27
Sickle knife

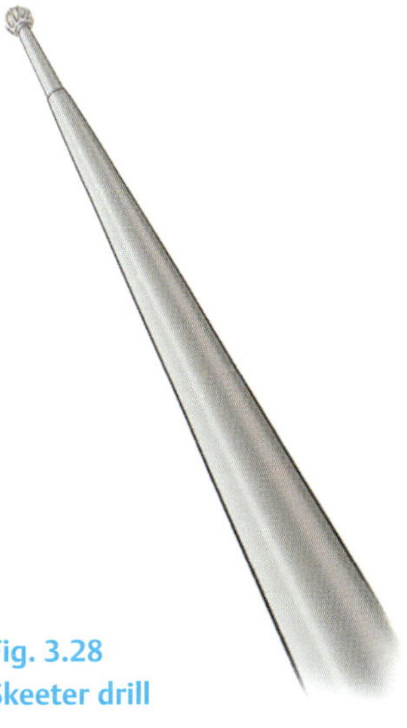

Fig. 3.28
Skeeter drill

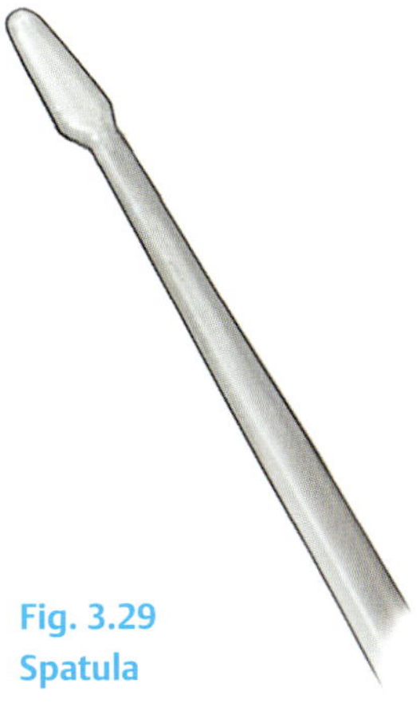

Fig. 3.29
Spatula

Surgical Monitoring

We employ two types of facial nerve monitoring. Mechanical pressure monitoring is used for stapes surgery and simple middle ear surgery without any risk of facial nerve injury. Electromyographic monitoring (NIM 3.0; Medtronic Xomed, Minneapolis, Minnesota, USA) is used for procedures where there are suspected facial nerve bony canal defects or middle ear malformation.

4

Management of Tympanic Membrane Abnormalities

4__Management of Tympanic Membrane Abnormalities

Our teaching hospital mainly uses a retroauricular approach, except for otosclerosis surgery, myringoplasty with xenografts for small accessible posterior or inferior perforations, and functional revision surgery.

A retroauricular approach provides better access to the anterior wall of the external auditory canal, the tympanic membrane, and the middle ear, and allows an unplanned transmastoid route. It also enables easy temporalis fascia or conchal cartilage graft harvesting.

Harvesting of Graft Materials

Temporalis Fascia

Retroauricular Skin Incision

After pulling up the upper part of the auricle, the subcutaneous skin layer is incised with a no. 25 scalpel blade, 5 mm above the auricular attachment and slightly posterior to the helix attachment.

The incision is made anteroposteriorly for the first 3 cm. It then curves inferiorly 1 cm parallel to the auricular fold, ending 1 cm above the mastoid tip, which has been previously palpated.

The posterior auricular muscle is cut and the auricle is detached anteriorly just before reaching the perichondrium of the external canal to expose the temporalis fascia area.

Fig. 4.1

Tip: The fact that the skin incision runs anterior to the level of the helix attachment allows good mobilization of the auricle and good exposure of the temporalis fascia, like opening a book to 180°, without any tissue tension in any plane. Pulling the skin up with a forceps enables three-dimensional dissection and access to the different tissue layers.

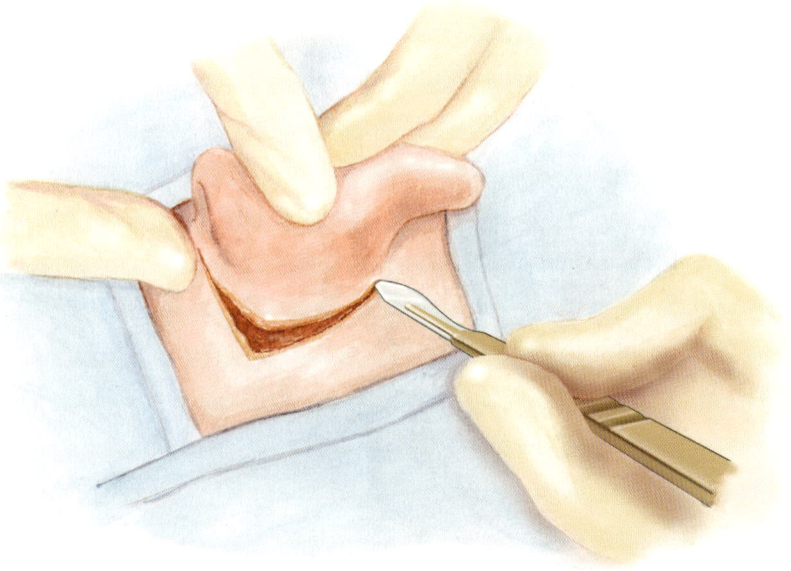

Fig. 4.1

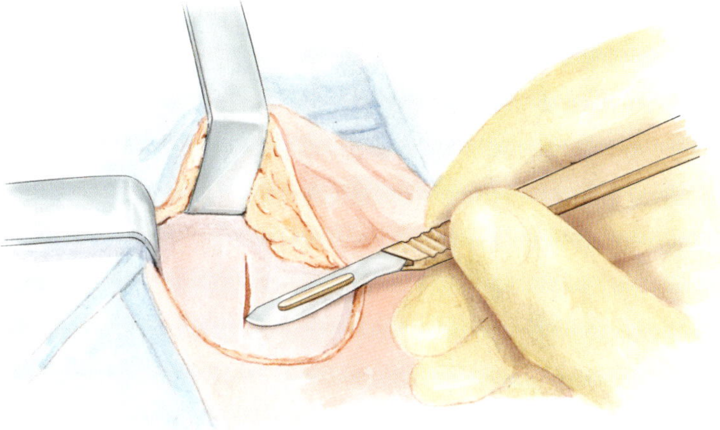

Fig. 4.2

Fascia Exposure and Incision

A self-retaining retractor held by the scrub nurse at an anterosuperior angle to the incision completely exposes the harvesting site.

The superficial fascia layer is removed and the fascia is cleaned with a Freer rugine. A 2-cm fascia incision is made with a no. 11 scalpel blade.

Fig. 4.2

Tip: Pulling the fascia up with a retractor helps to naturally find the layer that does not elevate but remains attached to the temporal muscle. Cleaning the fascia graft as much as possible before harvesting further facilitates fascia trimming.

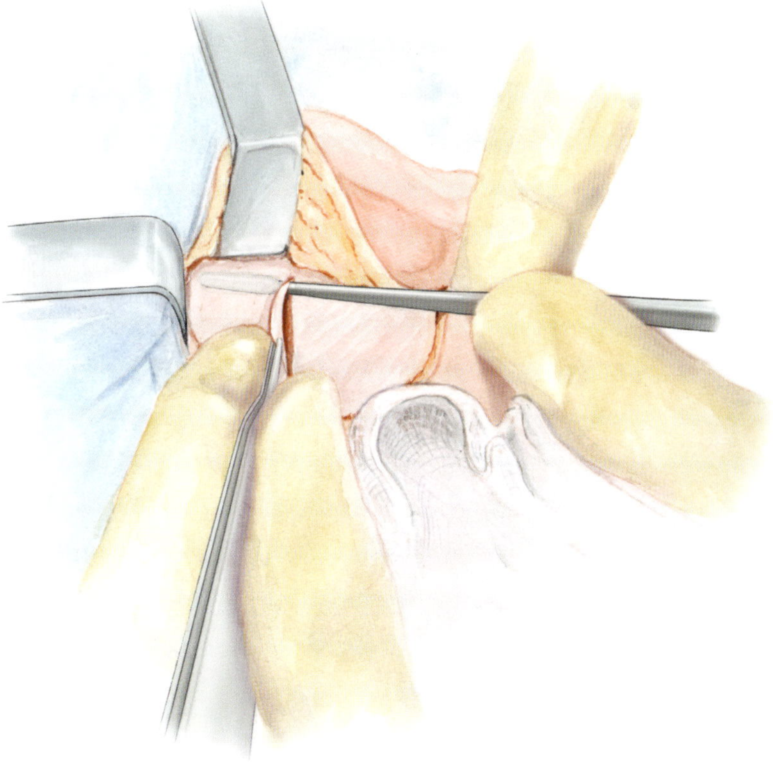

Fig. 4.3

Fascia Degloving

Elevation of the inferior side of the fascia from the temporal muscle is achieved with a Freer rugine.

Fig. 4.3

Fascia Removal

A rectangular fascia graft is excised off with blunt curved scissors, starting with an anterior and posterior incision and ending superiorly. The graft is removed with anatomical forceps.

Fig. 4.4

Hemostasis

Hemostasis of the muscle is performed very carefully due to the high risk of hematoma of the temporal region.

Fig. 4.5

Tip: The size of the fascia graft depends on the planned surgery. For a tympanoplasty, a graft between 1 and 1.5 cm^2 is sufficient. For mastoid cavity rehabilitation involving a large skin defect of the external auditory canal, harvest the largest graft possible. If second-stage surgery is planned, preserve fascia with easy access. In revision surgery, superior extension of the skin incision may be required to locate the temporalis fascia.

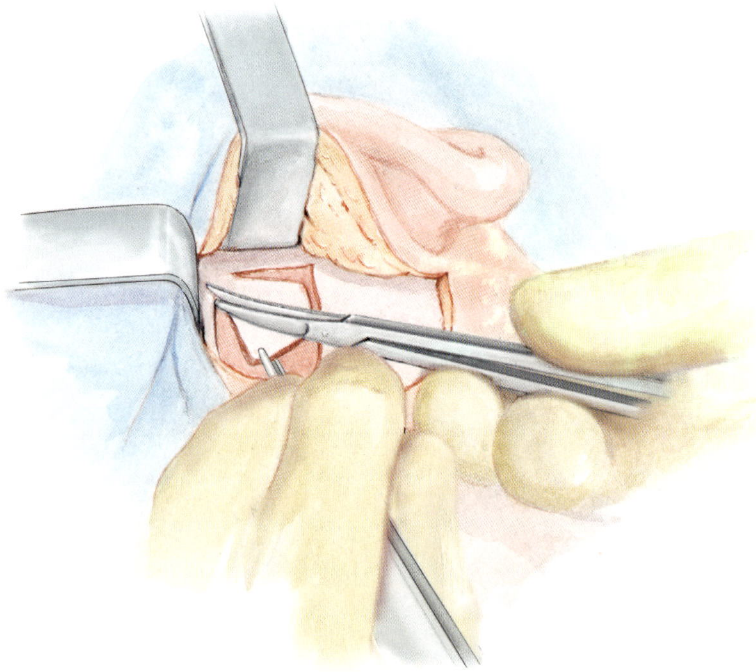

Fig. 4.4

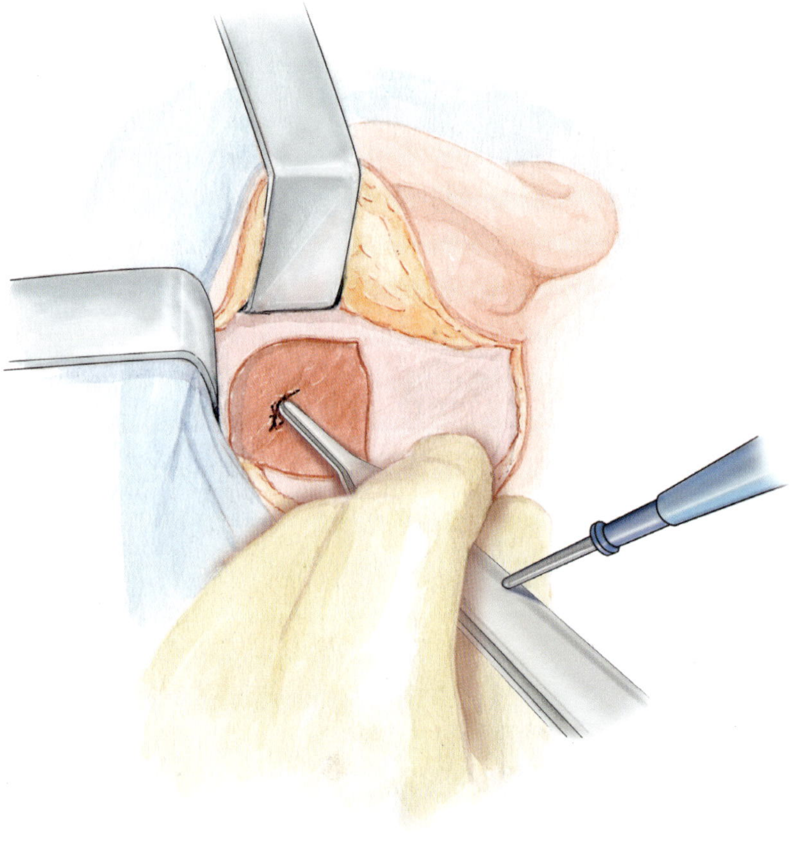

Fig. 4.5

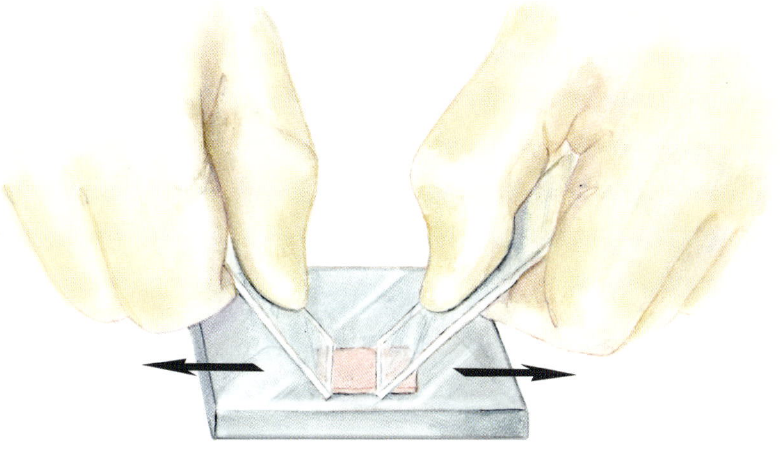

Fig. 4.6

Fascia Graft Preparation

The graft is cleaned and trimmed of residual muscle, superficial fascia, and fat using two histological glass slides, and flattened on a metallic sheet without being stretched. In the case of subtotal tympanoplasty, the graft is spread over a Perkins mold.

Fig. 4.6

Tip: Maintain the original size of the graft. Take care not to stretch the graft because it will shrink after placement and rehydration. Avoid contact of the graft with gloves and surgical fields to prevent contamination by microscopic foreign bodies, which can lead to myringitis

Tragal Cartilage–Perichondrium Graft

Tragal cartilage and perichondrium can be used for a simple cartilage graft, a perichondrial graft, or a cartilage–perichondrial graft.

Except in specific cases of footplate interposition, where we only use the posterior tragal perichondrium, the tragal cartilage is harvested with its perichondrium.

Preparation of the tragal support is always the same but the way it is used depends on surgical requirements.

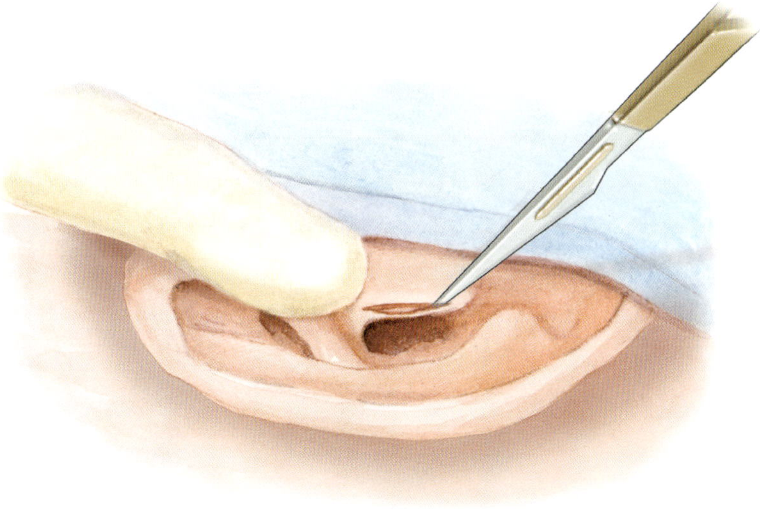

Fig. 4.7

Skin Incision

After infiltration of lidocaine and epinephrine, a 1.5-cm skin incision is made on the dome of the tragal cartilage with a no. 11 scalpel blade. The cartilage edge lies just beneath the incision.

Fig. 4.7

Tip: Note the position of the finger on the illustration. This facilitates the incision under the dome edge. It also helps cosmetically.

Graft Exposure

The subcutaneous tissue is dissected posteriorly and anteriorly from the perichondrium using opening movements of pointed curved scissors over the entire surface of the cartilage. Anatomical forceps help to elevate the skin and improve the view.

Graft Excision

The cartilage is pulled in a superior direction with anatomical forceps to incise the cartilage inferiorly with blunt curved scissors. An anterior incision is made as deep as possible.

Fig. 4.8

Finally, a superior incision is made.

Fig. 4.9

Removing the entire cartilage dome improves the esthetic appearance. Bleeding is controlled, and the skin incision is closed with fibrin glue or stitches.

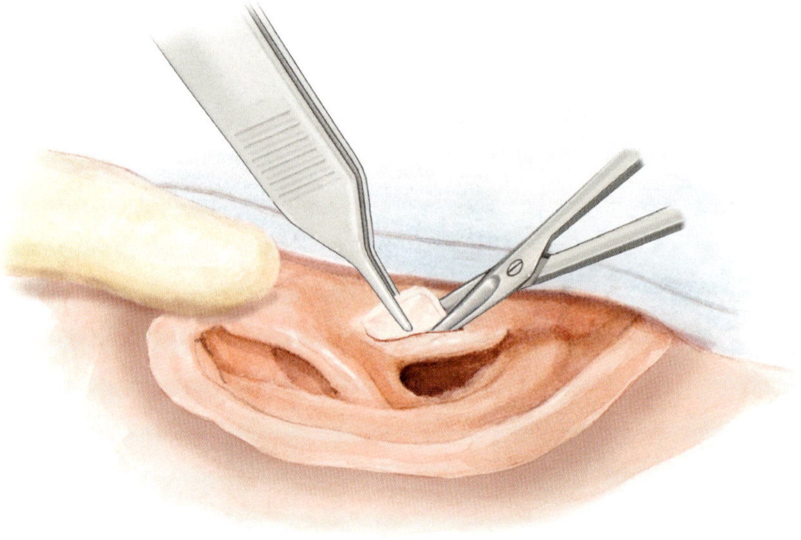

Fig. 4.8

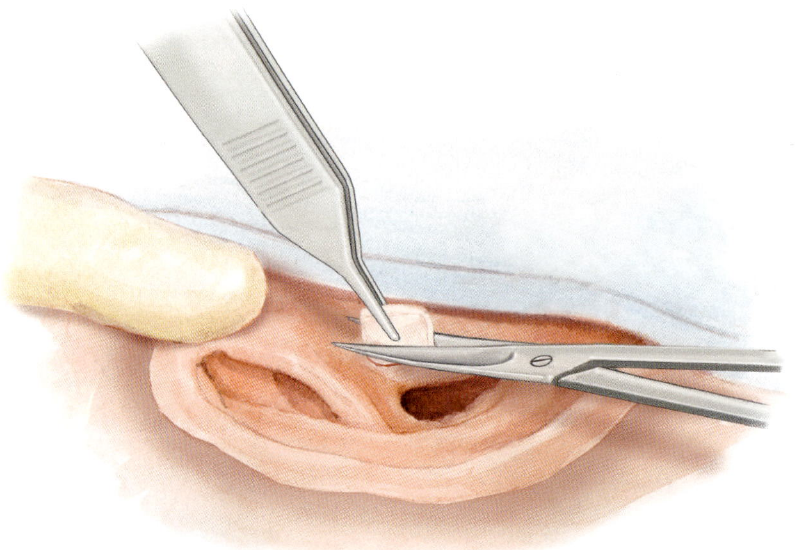

Fig. 4.9

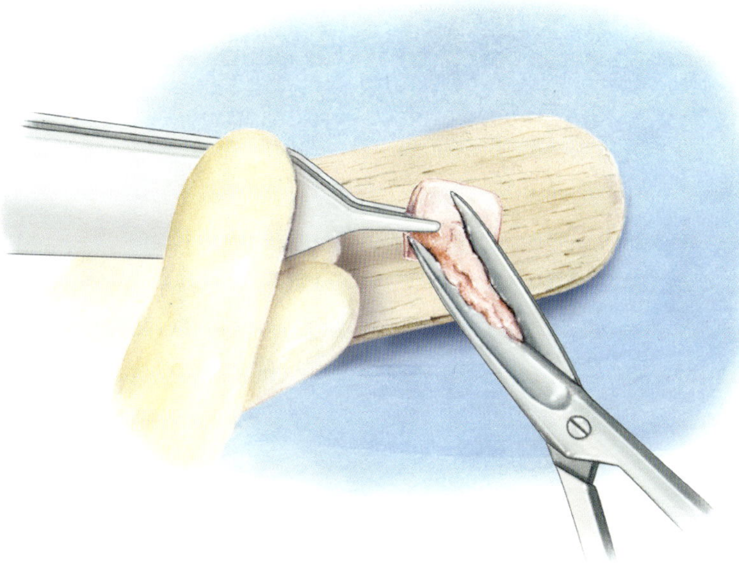

Fig. 4.10

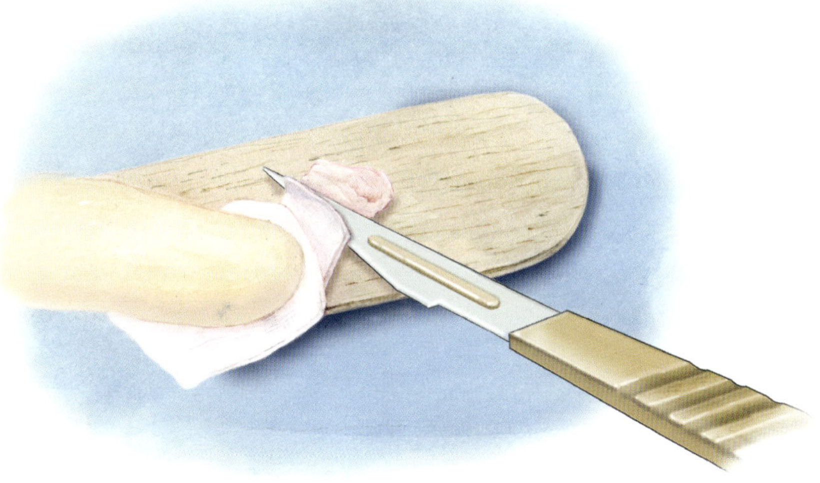

Fig. 4.11

Perichondrium Elevation and Cleaning

The tragus is fixed with a small compress under the thumb on a metallic sheet or a wooden tongue depressor.

For attic bony defect reconstruction or posterior tympanic cartilage reconstruction, the anterior perichondrium is detached with a flap knife from the medial cutting edge to the dome of the cartilage (like opening the front page of a book). The posterior perichondrium remains intact.

The anterior perichondrium is cleaned of the residual subcutaneous tissue using blunt curved scissors. This is called a cartilage–perichondrium graft.

For other uses (total tympanoplasty, bony defect reconstruction, prosthesis interposition, ossiculoplasty), the anterior and posterior perichondria are separated from the cartilage en bloc. The perichondrium is dried out in a press. The cartilage is preserved in a humid compress.

Fig. 4.10

Tip: A wooden tongue depressor helps to keep the graft from sliding and is easy to handle.

Cartilage Refinement

On a wooden tongue depressor, the cartilage, with or without the perichondrium, is refined using a no. 11 scalpel blade.

The cartilage is preserved for further processing depending on its use.

Fig. 4.11

Cartilage Chips

The cartilage can be cut into chips for tympanic reconstruction or prosthesis interposition, into small pieces for ossiculoplasty, into large pieces for bony defect reconstruction, and left en bloc for posterior tympanic reconstruction. **Fig. 4.12**

Everything except the perichondrium is placed in a compress soaked with physiological saline solution.

Tip: These different applications should be prepared just before starting reconstruction.

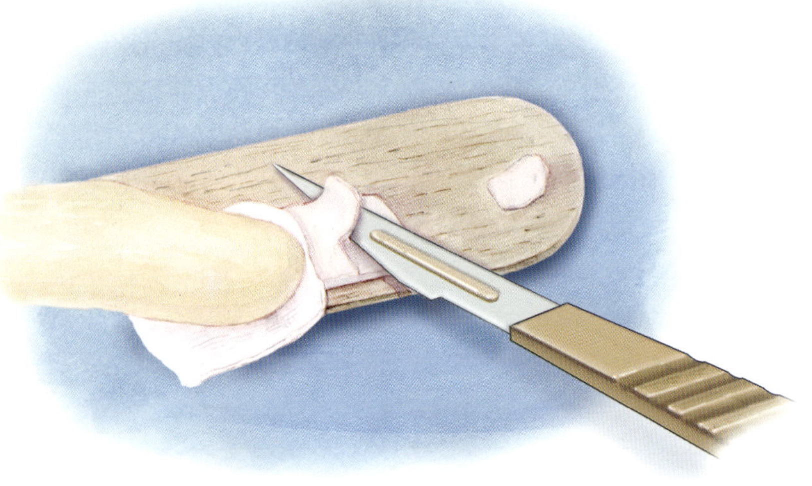

Fig. 4.12

Conchal Cartilage Graft

The advantage of conchal cartilage over tragal cartilage is the availability of a larger surface area. However, conchal cartilage perichondrium is of poor quality and cannot generally be used. For tympanic reconstruction, tragal cartilage is therefore preferred.

Cartilage Exposition

After dissection and elevation of the subcutaneous tissue and postauricular muscle using pointed curved scissors, the conchal cartilage eminence is exposed by means of the retroauricular incision. **Fig. 4.13**

Tip: Placing a finger in the concha stabilizes the dissection, thus avoiding puncture of the conchal skin.

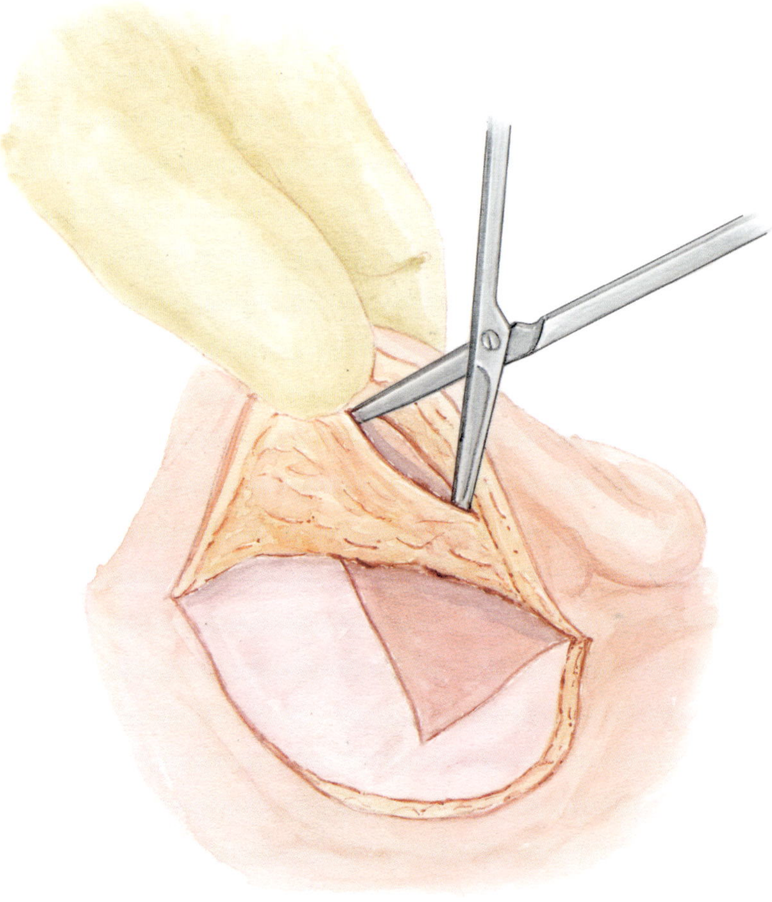

Fig. 4.13

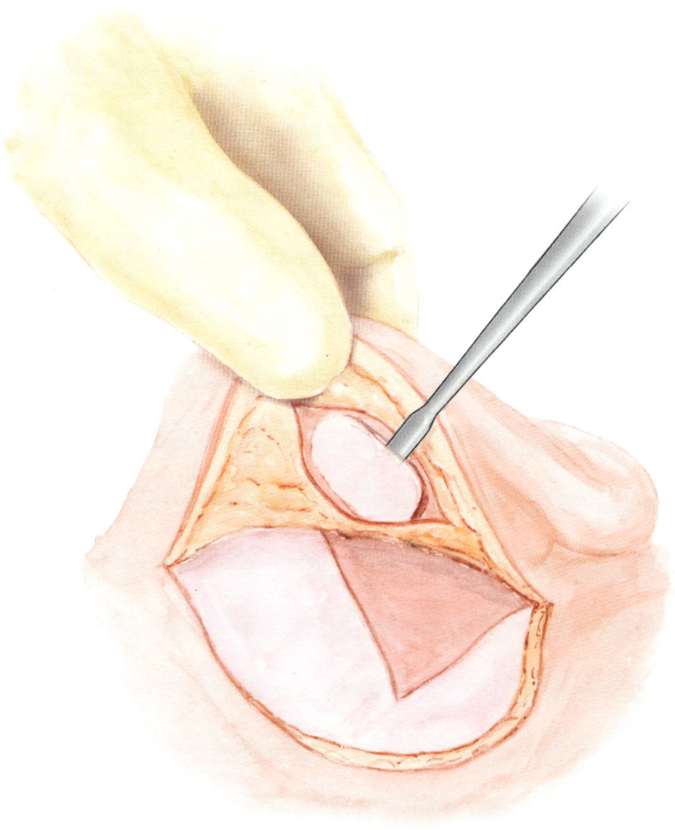

Fig. 4.14

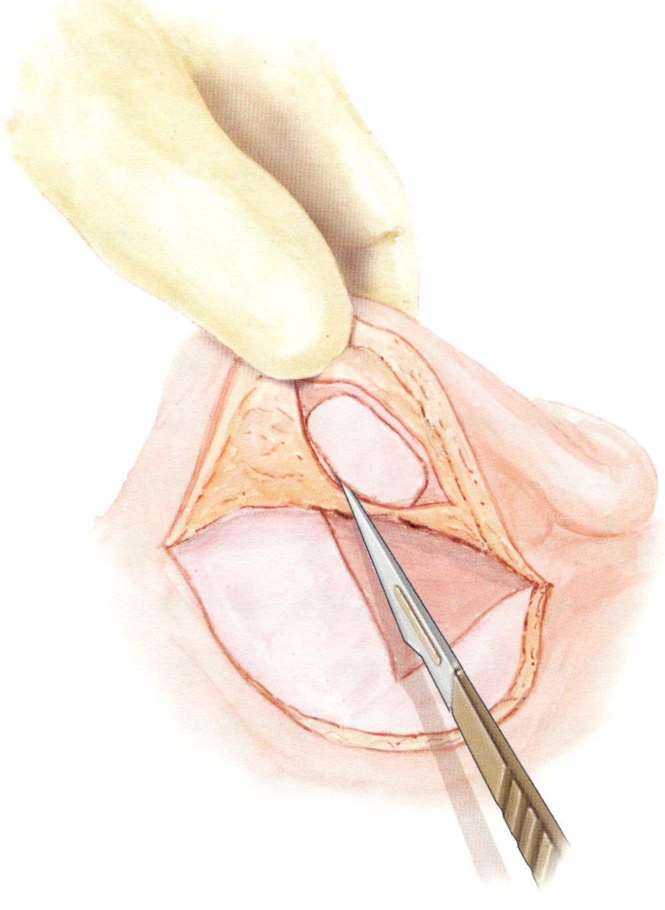

Fig. 4.15

Cartilage Incision

The perichondrium and cartilage are incised superiorly using a no. 11 scalpel blade.

The perichondrium and cartilage are held with anatomical forceps, and the cartilage is elevated from the anterior tissue with the periosteal elevator.

Fig. 4.14

Cartilage Excision

When the elevated surface area is sufficient, lateral and inferior incisions are made using blunt scissors or a scalpel blade.

Fig. 4.15

On a wooden tongue depressor, the posterior perichondrium is cleaned of residual subcutaneous tissue using blunt curved scissors. The perichondrium can also be removed but cannot usually be used because of its poor quality. Subcutaneous tissue above the harvesting site must be sutured.

Fatty Tissue Graft

For fatty tissue myringoplasty, fat can be harvested from the ear lobe or the abdomen (incision in the umbilicus or any previous incision site).

The ear lobe is infiltrated with lidocaine and epinephrine. A skin incision is made on the posterior side of the edge of the lobe. The fat is dissected using pointed curved scissors, taking care not to penetrate the anterior or posterior skin.

Fig. 4.16

The incision is closed using fibrin glue or stitches. The fat is preserved in a disinfectant solution.

Skin Graft

When a skin graft is required for partial external auditory canal reconstruction, the harvest graft is taken from the posterior edge of the retroauricular incision, mostly inferiorly, where there is no hair. The strip is between 5 and 7 mm in width, 2 cm in length, and as thin as possible.

Fig. 4.17

The skin graft is preserved flat in a compress, humidified with physiological saline solution, or flattened in a press.

If a larger graft is required, the skin is harvested with a dermatome from the inner biceps.

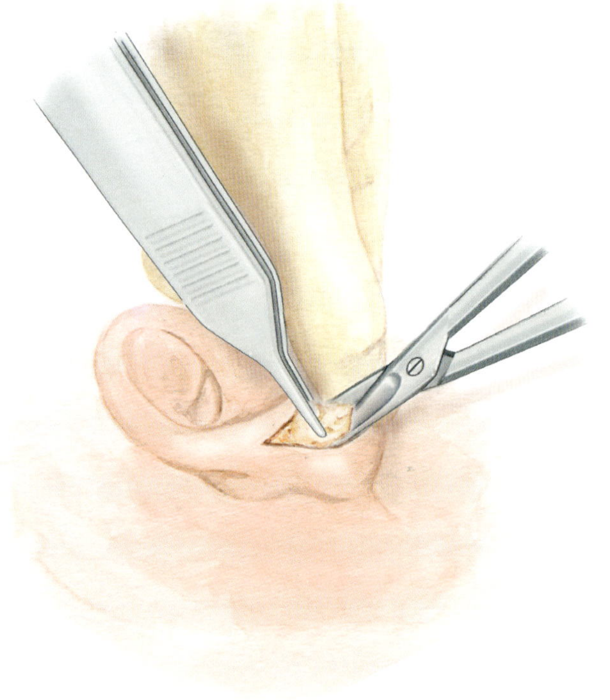

Fig. 4.16

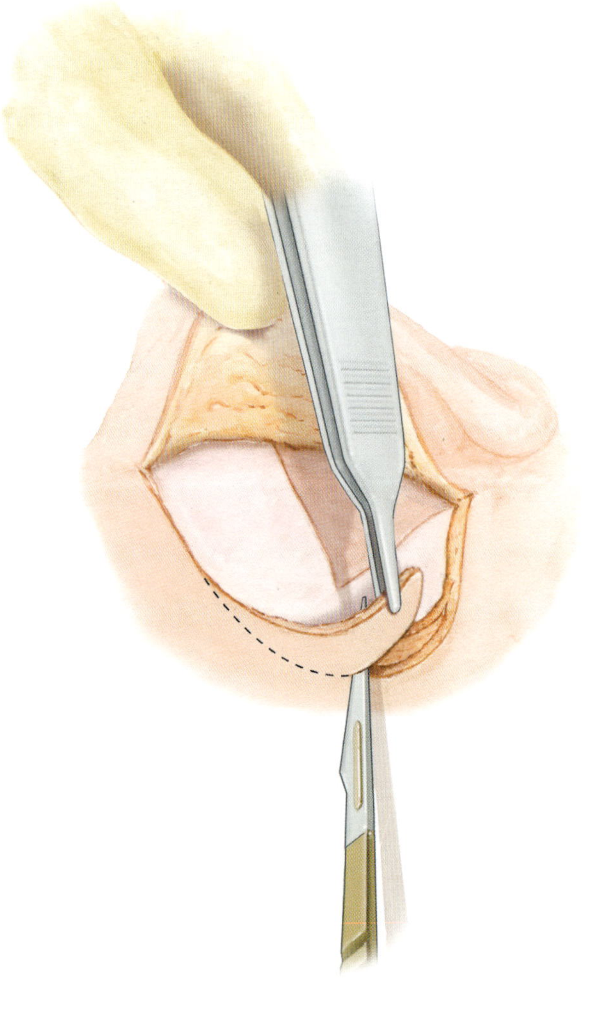

Fig. 4.17

Tympanic Membrane Approaches

Retroauricular Approach

The retroauricular approach is our preferred option because it provides better access to the anterior tympanum and protympanic region. It allows easy harvesting of the temporalis fascia and conchal cartilage, and unplanned implementation of the transmastoid approach.

Tip: Take the time to examine the skin quality properly, as well as the tympanic membrane and the canal anatomy. This helps in planning further skin incisions.

Transcanal Approach

A transcanal approach is used in the majority of stapes surgery, functional revision surgery, explorative surgery for conductive deafness with an intact eardrum, and myringoplasty with xenografts for otoscopically confirmed small posteroinferior perforation.

Nasal Speculum

A nasal speculum is used at the beginning of surgery to evaluate the meatal and tympanic membrane anatomy and skin quality as well as to clean and rinse with saline solution.

Advantages of the nasal speculum are that it makes it easy to change the operative field of vision and adapts to all canal diameters. The disadvantage is the sacrifice of the surgeon's second hand

Fig. 4.18

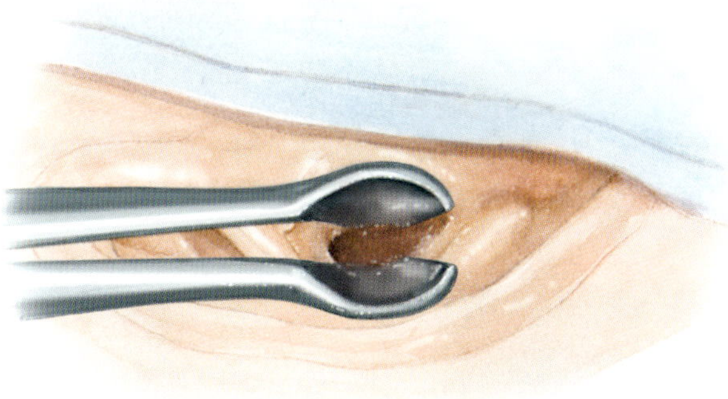

Fig. 4.18

Tip: Holding the nasal speculum in the palm of the hand is more comfortable.

The Portmann Fixed Ear Speculum

For a transcanal approach, when no great change in the angle of visualization is required, a fixed speculum is used. The Portmann speculum allows the soft external auditory canal to be extended as far as possible. The holder arm is fixed to the operating table and centered on the canal.

Fig. 4.19

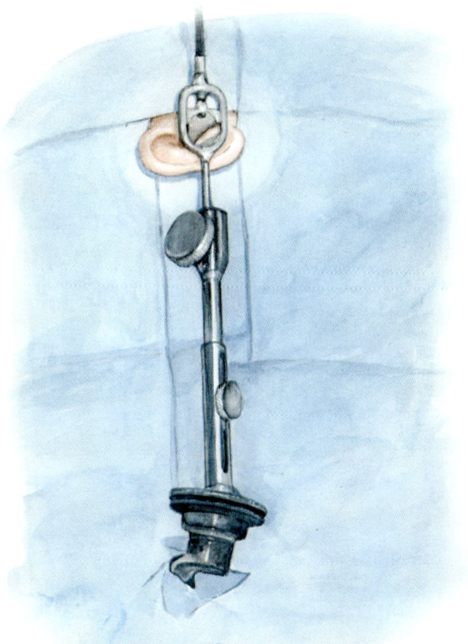

Fig. 4.19

Tip: After placement, do not touch the speculum change the position of the table instead.

Skin Incision

See Retroauricular Skin Incision, p. 18

Fig. 4.20

Musculoperiosteal Flap

The self-retaining retractor is utilized to pull up the skin flap. Using electrocautery, the superior incision of the musculoperiosteal flap starts anteriorly at the level of the temporal line, running toward the posterior skin incision. Inferiorly, it ends at the inferior edge of the external auditory canal, creating an anteriorly based isoscel triangle centered on the inferior edge of the Henle spine.

Fig. 4.21

For mastoidectomy, the musculoperiosteal flap is enlarged into a trapezium to expose the mastoid process.

Tip: Place your finger in the meatus it helps to localize the external auditory canal and to center the musculoperiosteal flap. Mark the temporal line to determine the superior limit of the flap. Palpate the mastoid tip to avoid the risk of damaging the facial nerve in the stylomastoid area, especially in children.

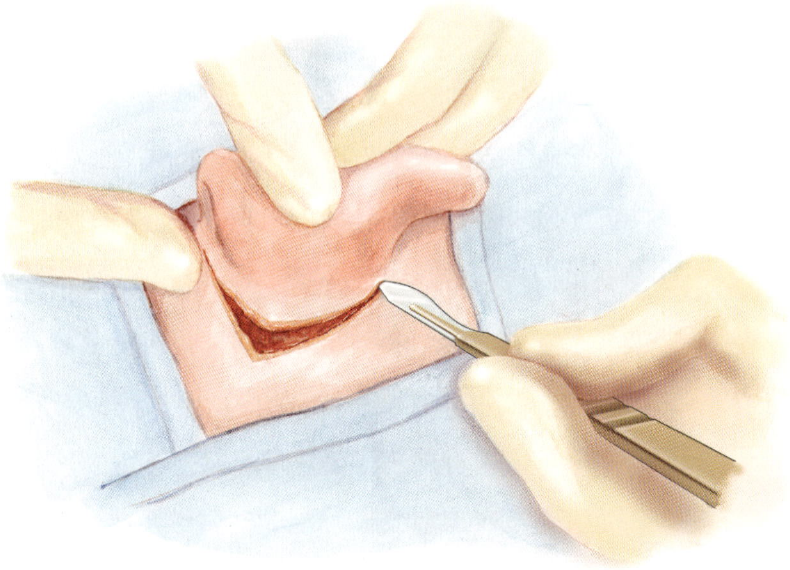

Fig. 4.20

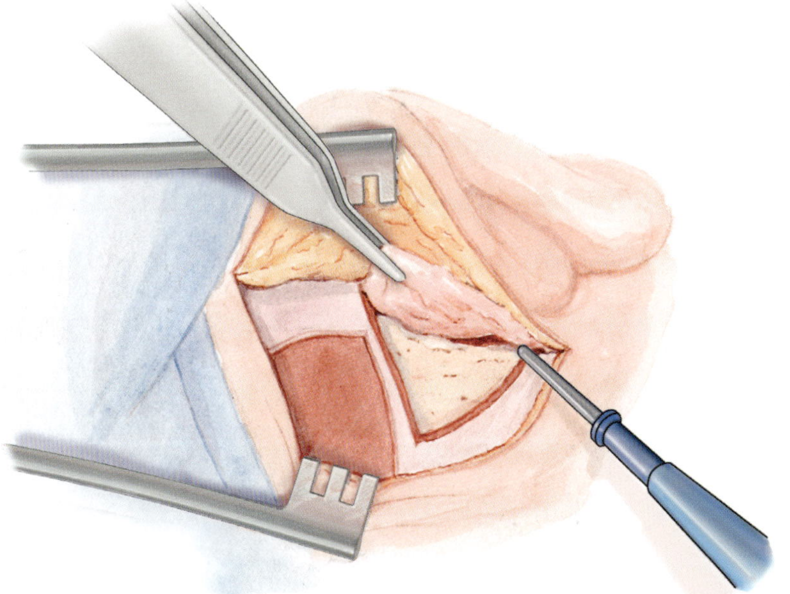

Fig. 4.21

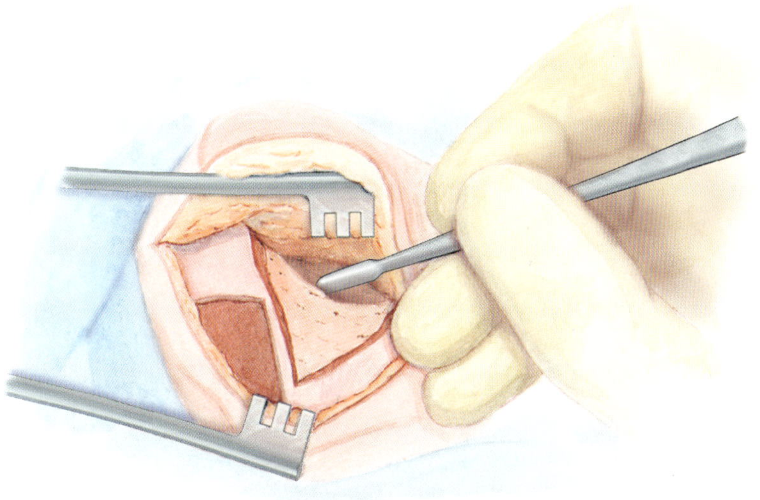

Fig. 4.22

Flap Elevation

The flap is elevated up to the meatus with a periosteal elevator, and the retractor is repositioned to hold both flaps.

The posterior skin of the external auditory canal is detached using a raspatory superiorly and inferiorly from 10 to 4 o'clock. Opening the retractor gently aids a natural degloving, except in revision surgery, where the skin is too fragile.

Fig. 4.22

Meatal Skin Counterincision

Using a no. 11 scalpel, a circumferential incision of the posterior canal skin is made in the center of the canal and first followed inferiorly. This allows localization of the tympanic membrane through the incision. The inferior lateral incision is continued for ± 1 cm.

Fig. 4,23

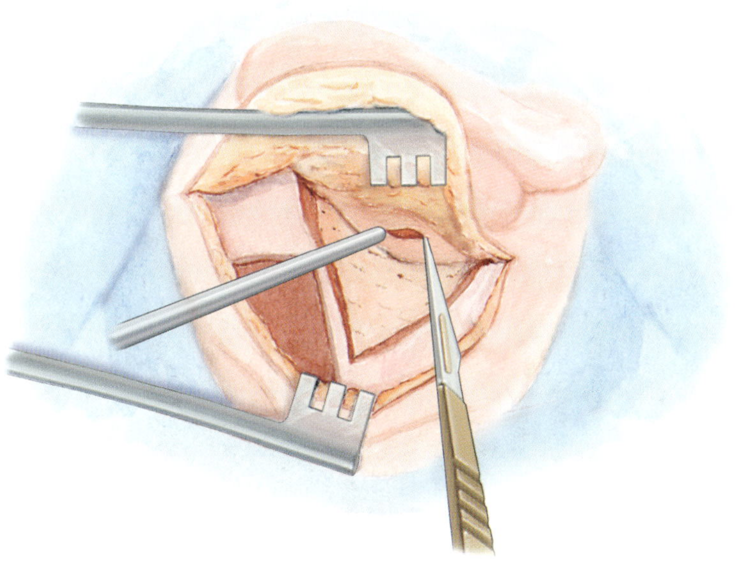

Fig. 4.23

Vascular Strip

The superior part of the circumferential incision and the superior lateral incision are then completed. A laterally based meatal skin flap, known as a posterior vascular strip, is obtained.

Fig. 4.24

Incision Distance

The distance of the circumferential incision depends on the type of tympanoplasty:

For subtotal perforation, the incision is located as close as possible to the ear drum (A).

If the tympanic membrane is intact, or in other types of perforation or pathology, the incision is located approximately 8 mm from the ear drum or just above the external ear canal pathology (B).

For canal wall down tympanoplasty, the incision is located approximately 5 mm below the inferior edge of the conchal cartilage, and the lateral incision is shorter (C).

Fig. 4.25

Tip: Application of small-diameter (to prevent tearing) microsuction to the meatal skin helps to tighten the skin for easier incision.

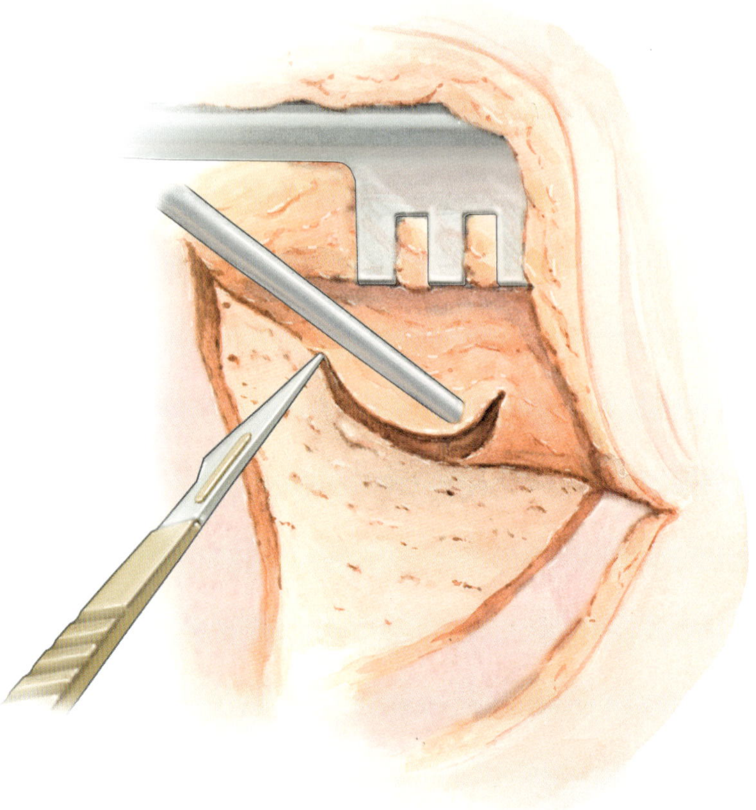

Fig. 4.24

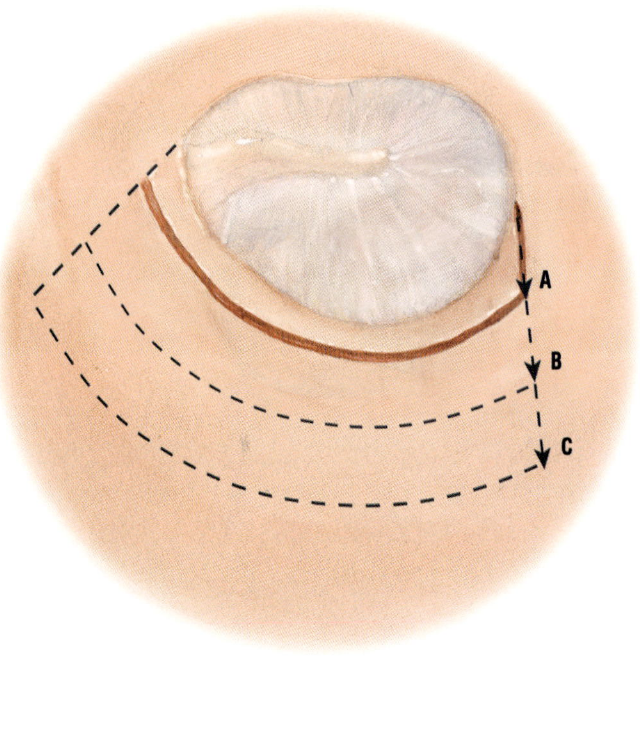

Fig. 4.25

Vascular Strip Elevation

A string or strip of gauze is pushed into the external canal and pulled out through the incision of the laterally based skin flap.

Fig. 4.26

Optimal Exposure

The string is attached to the surgical field with a clamp, and a self-retaining retractor is used to hold the musculoperiosteal and skin flaps in place. Good exposure is required to visualize the anterior wall and ensure an unimpaired view of the tympanic membrane.

Fig. 4.27

Tip: To achieve safe and adequate elevation of the laterally based skin flap, the strip needs to be as flat as possible. Placement of a self-retaining retractor on the strip helps it not to slide. If the vascular strip remains elevated and exposure is sufficient, the string is not necessary.

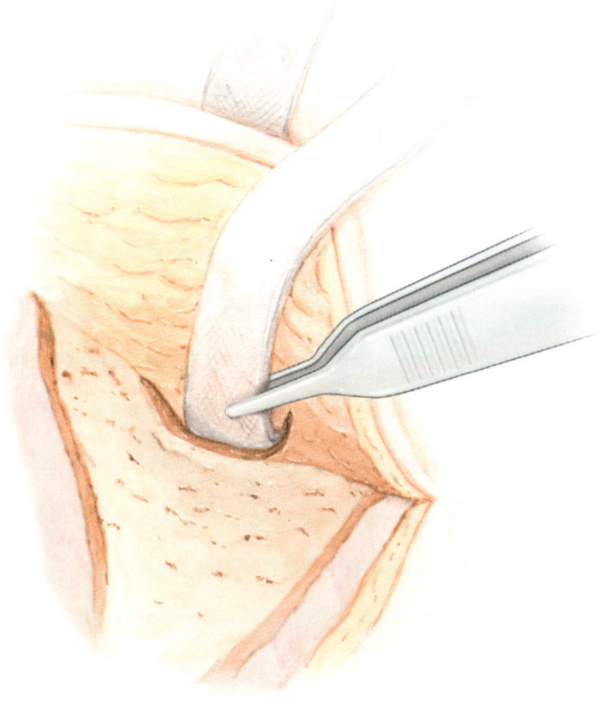

Fig. 4.26

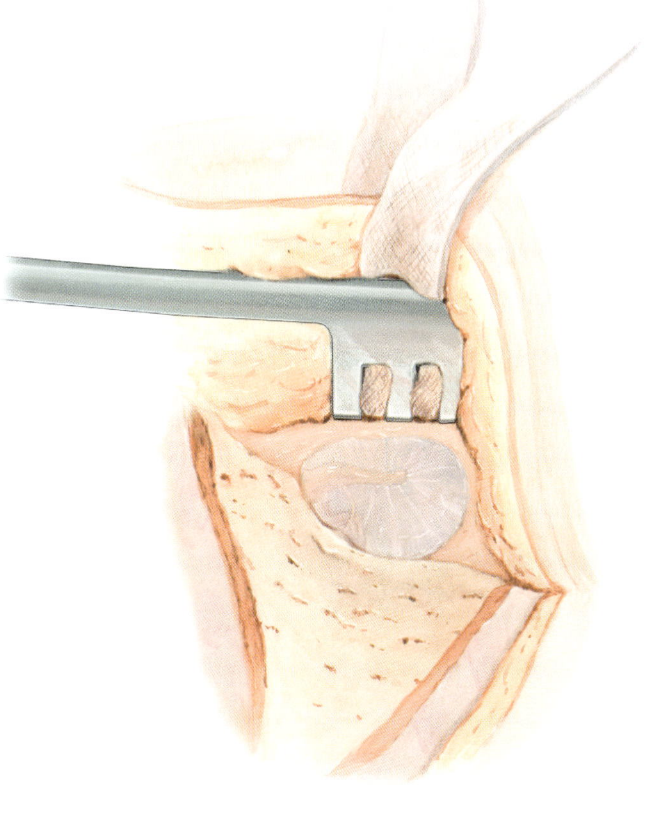

Fig. 4.27

Difficult Retroauricular Approaches

To ensure a satisfactory surgical procedure, it is absolutely vital to have a good enough view of the annulus and the tympanic perforation. Bulges of the posterior bony canal, protrusions of the anterior bony canal, and prominent bony sutures are frequent. In such cases, a canaloplasty should be performed by drilling the wall in the following order: posterior, inferior, superior, anterior.

Protrusion of the Posterior Bony Canal Wall

Henle Spine Protrusion

A protruding Henle spine is removed using a cutting burr or chisel.

Drilling the posterior bony canal wall may be sufficient to expose the anterior annulus. Using a large cutting burr, drilling is started laterally parallel to the tympanic membrane, progressing medially until the anterior annulus is visualized. Protecting the skin flap with Merocel (Merocel, Minneapolis, Minnesota, USA) or an aluminum sheet may be necessary. If mastoid cells are exposed, they must be closed off with bone pâté or wax, soft tissue, or a cartilage graft to avoid iatrogenic cholesteatoma.

Fig. 4.28

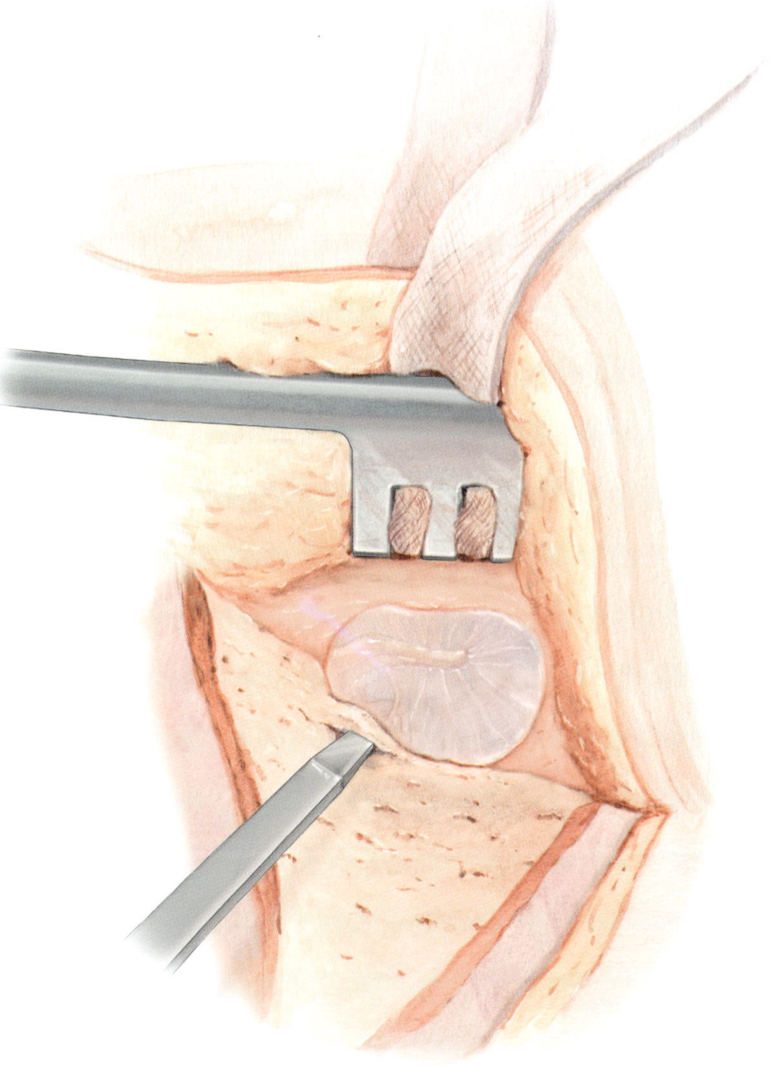

Fig. 4.28

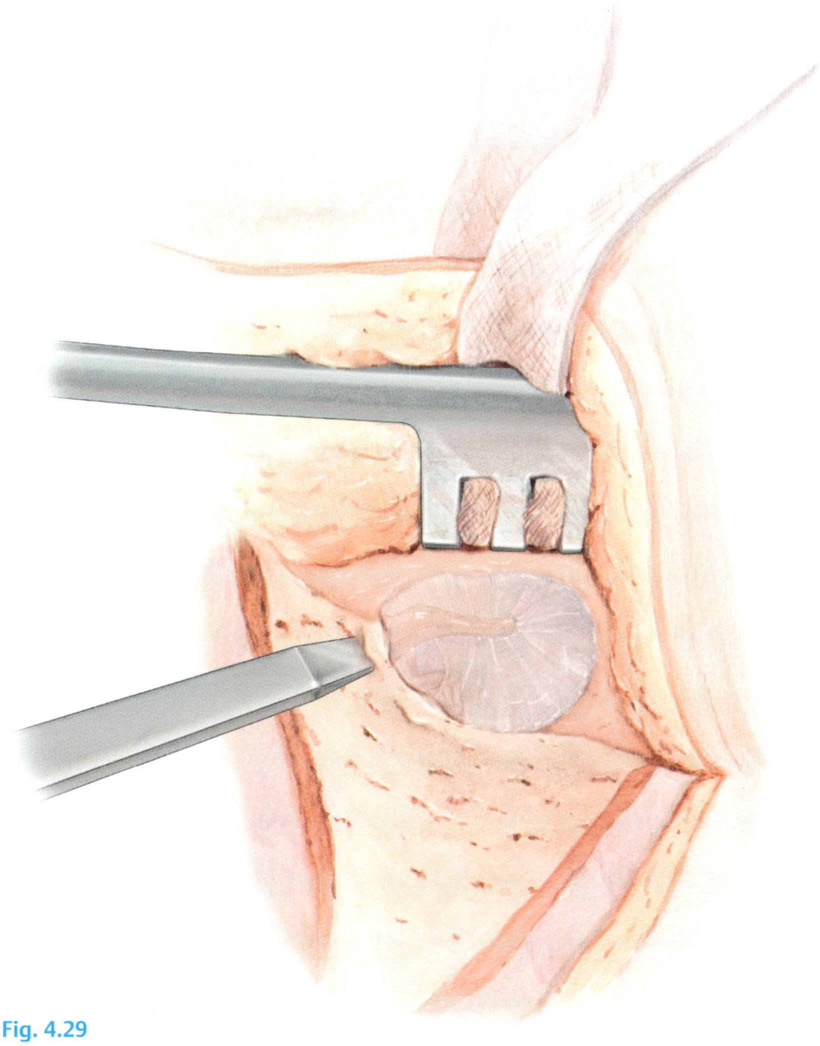

Fig. 4.29

Protrusion of the Bony Sutures

Bony Suture Excision

Detachment of the skin from the tympanosquamous and/or tympanomastoid suture may require difficult dissection of adhesions between the suture and the bony canal using electrocautery or a no. 11 scalpel. Once free of the skin, the suture is removed using a cutting or diamond burr or a small chisel. When drilling, the skin flaps must be completely covered with a Merocel, Silastic (Dow Corning, Midland, Michigan, USA), or aluminum sheet (obtained from the surgical thread packaging) to avoid damage. Drilling or removing sutures near the short process of the malleus is dangerous.

Fig. 4.29

Tip: Do not use cutting burrs near the tympanic membrane, and adjust your burr diameter to maintain a good view. Irrigate abundantly.

Anterior Canal Wall Protrusion

Anterior Meatal Skin Flap

This technique is a slight variant of the posterior vascular strip technique described by Sheehy and Patterson (1967).

A medial blind circumferential skin incision is made just above the annulus if possible, using a round knife or no. 11 scalpel blade. A lateral circumferential skin incision is then made with a no. 11 scalpel blade 2–3 mm above the protrusion. The meatal skin is first elevated from the bone a few millimeters above the annulus along the circumferential incision, then pushed gradually from inferior to superior. The skin is completely removed and kept flat in gauze soaked in physiological saline solution or in a press.
Fig. 4.30

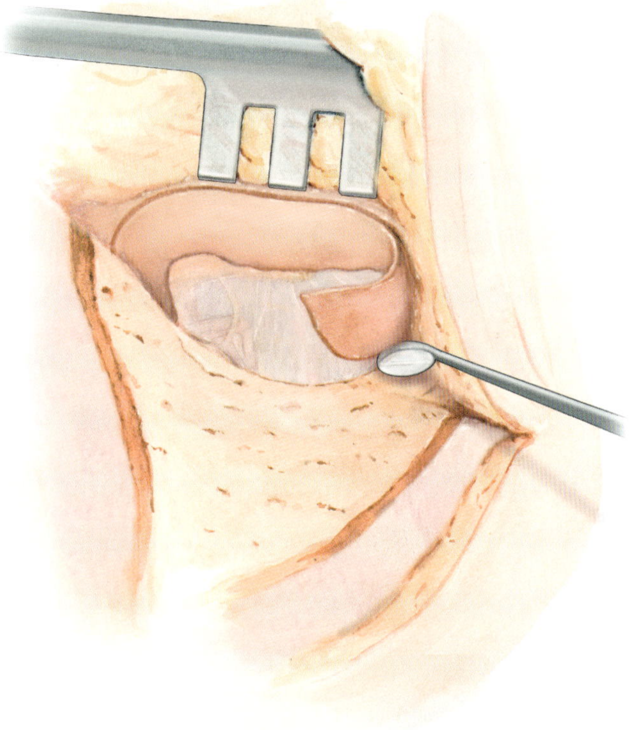

Fig. 4.30

Anterior Bony Wall Drilling

The tympanic membrane is protected with Merocel or an aluminum sheet. Using a relatively large cutting burr, drilling is started laterally, moving parallel to the tympanic membrane, advancing medially. The size of the burr is gradually reduced and a diamond burr or curette is used just above the tympanic membrane. Care must be taken not to penetrate the temporomandibular joint or touch the short process of the malleus.
Fig. 4.31

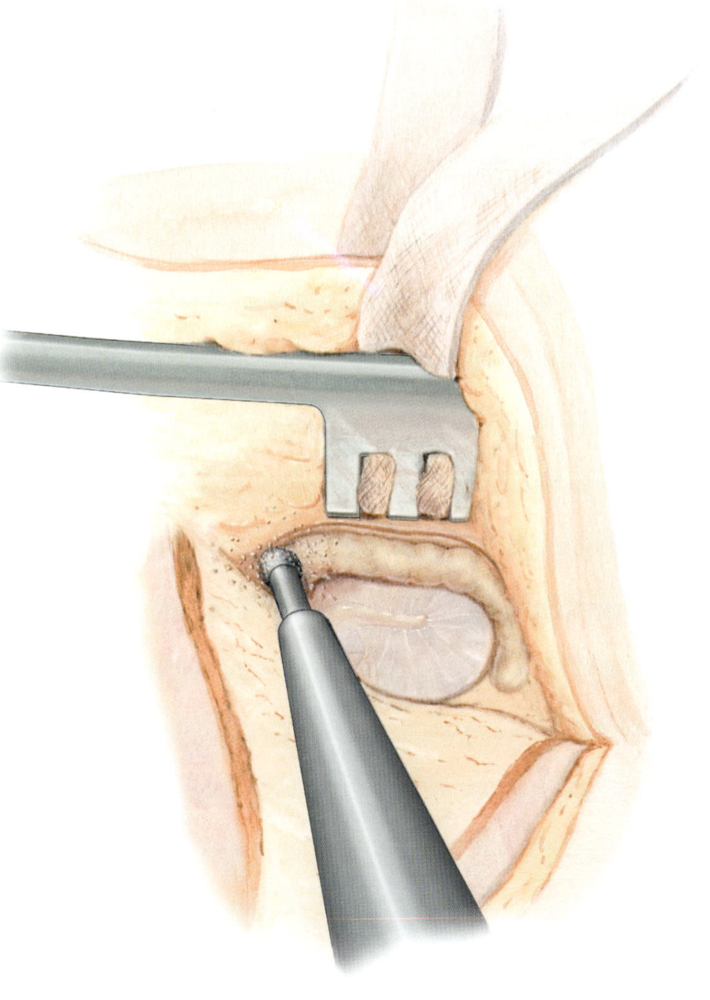

Fig. 4.31

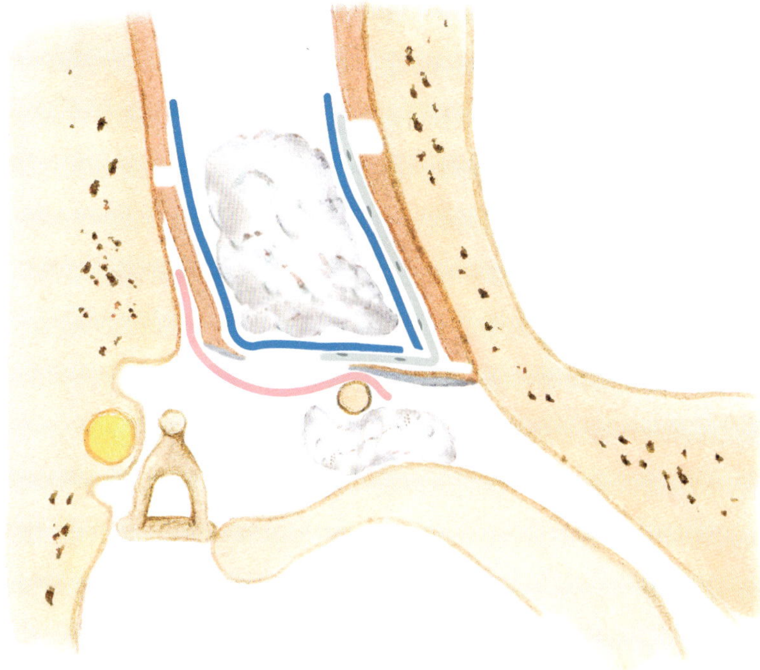

Fig. 4.32

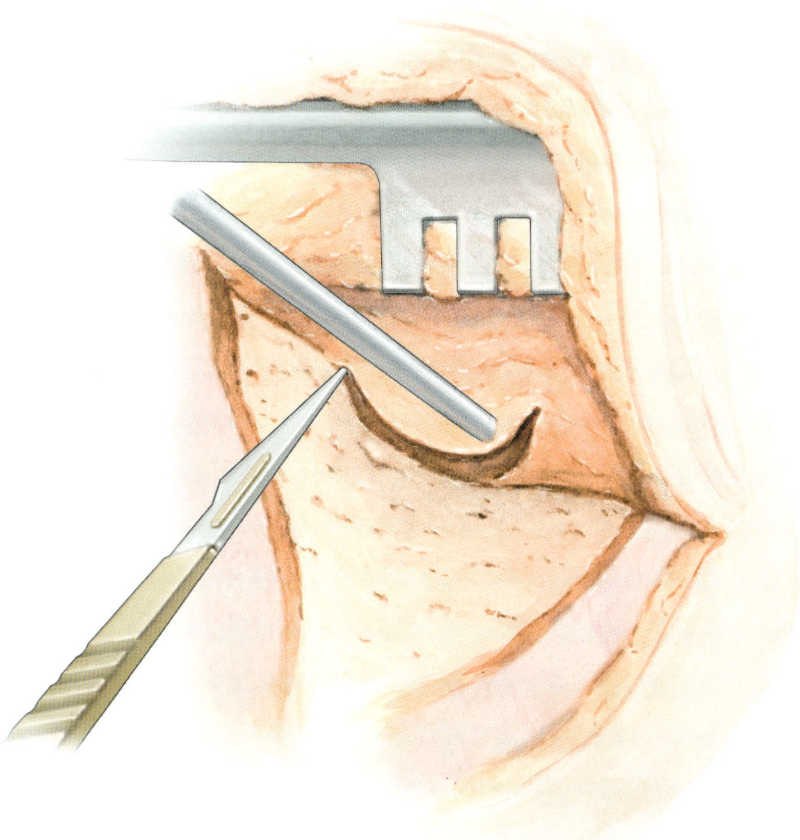

Fig. 4.33

Anterior Skin Flap Repositioning
After tympanoplasty, the skin flap is repositioned and glued. Packing with Epifilm improves healing (see Packing, p. 50).

Fig. 4.32

Tip: Be sure that the flap is repositioned on the right side. If the skin flap is insufficient or too damaged, use a free skin graft (see Skin Graft, p. 26).

Tympanic Membrane Perforations

Posteroinferior Perforation

Meatal Skin Counterincision
A circumferential incision of the laterally based meatal skin flap is made approximately 8 mm from the ear drum.

Fig. 4.33

Optimal Exposure
The vascular strip is elevated with a strip of gauze and a self-retaining retractor is used to hold the musculoperiosteal and skin flaps in place (see Figs. 4.25, 4.26).

Excision of the Perforation Edge
Using a sickle knife, the edge of the perforation is incised through all three layers of the eardrum all around the circumference of the perforation.

Fig. 4.34

Edge Removal
The edge is removed with microforceps, moving from the cutting point to the center of the perforation. Care is taken not to remove too much of the lamina propria.

In the case of tympanosclerotic plaques, the epithelium is scratched from the edge.

Fig. 4.35

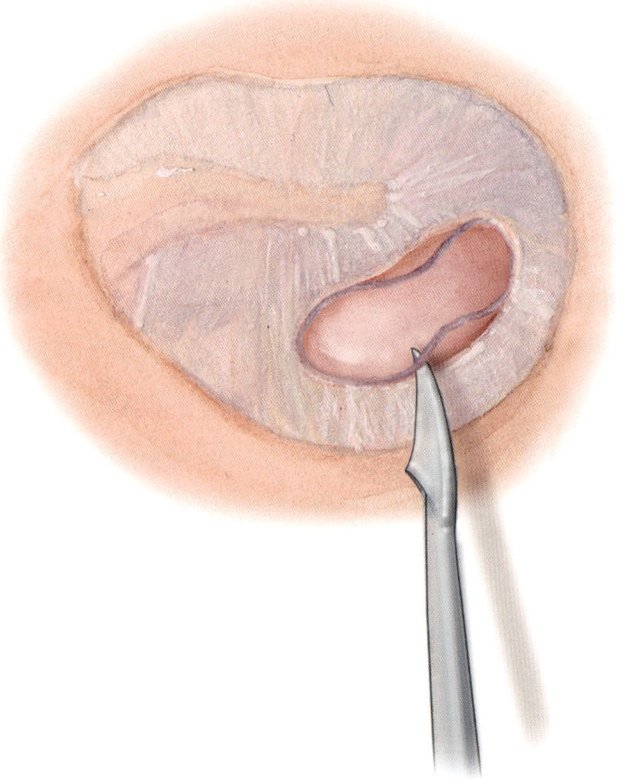

Fig. 4.34

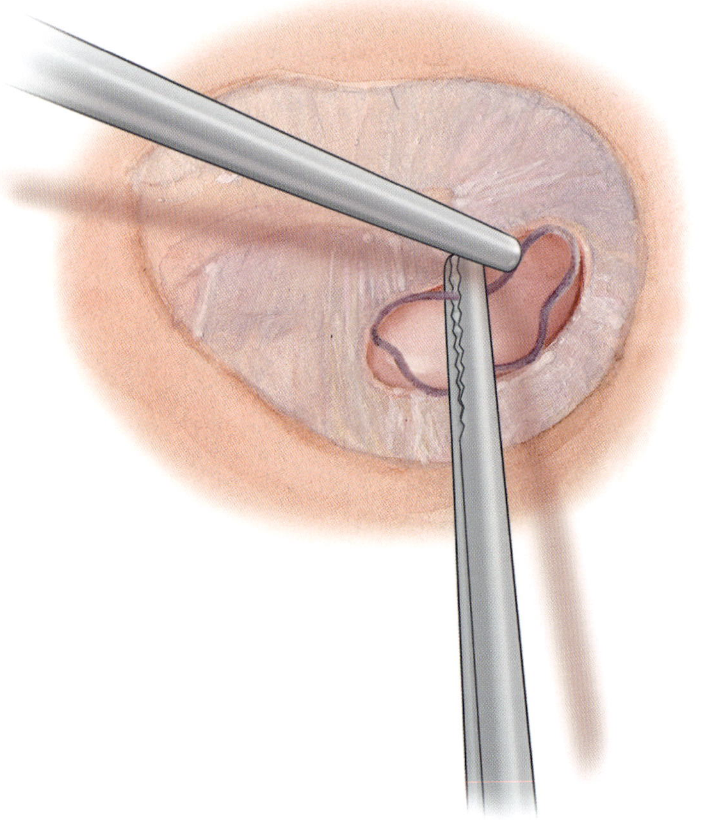

Fig. 4.35

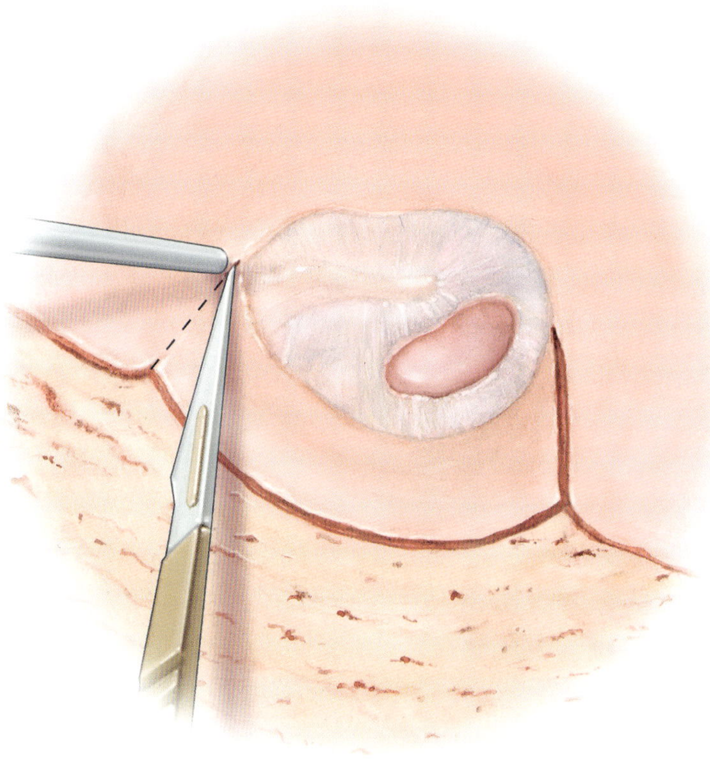

Fig. 4.36

Tympanomeatal Flap Incision

A superior lateral incision is made from the superior corner of the circumferential incision to just above the short process of the malleus.

An inferior lateral incision is made from 2–3 mm above the annulus to the anterior level of the perforation. These incisions are performed with a no. 11 scalpel.

Fig. 4.36

Tip: Use of a no. 11 scalpel blade allows a straight incision to be made, prevents skin tearing, and reduces bleeding.

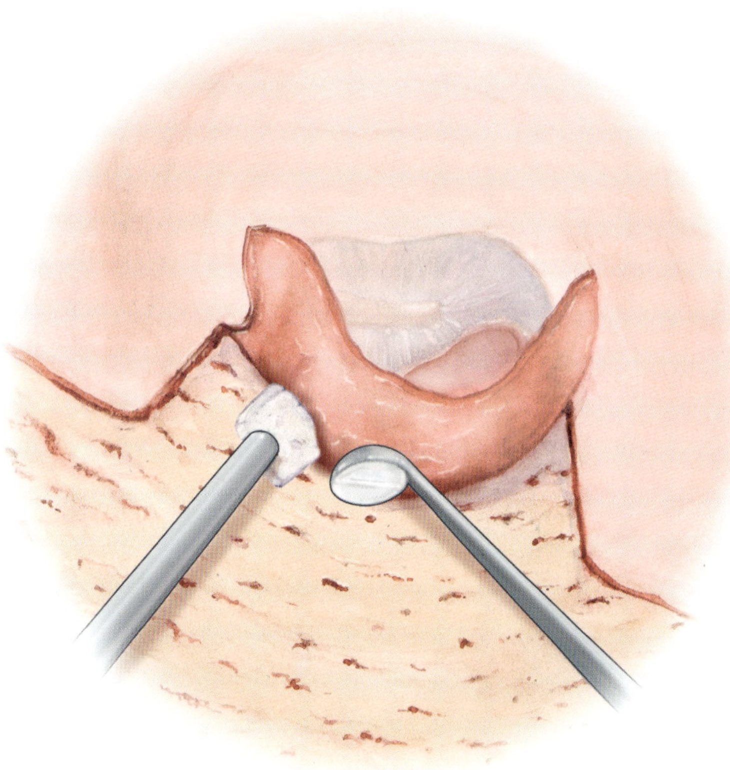

Fig. 4.37

Tympanomeatal Flap Elevation

The meatal skin is elevated toward the fibrous annulus with a small round knife. Microsuction is performed with a small piece of Merocel or a cotton ball soaked in 1% lidocaine with 5 µg/mL epinephrine to protect the fragile skin and reduce bleeding.

Fig. 4.37

Fibrous Annulus Dislocation
With a needle or sickle knife, the fibrous annulus is dislocated from its sulcus, beginning at the chordal eminence, being especially careful around the chorda tympani. The middle ear mucosa must be incised to enter the middle ear cavity.
Fig. 4.38

Tympanic Membrane Dislocation
When the opening is large enough, a flap knife or dissector-elevator is inserted and the fibrous annulus inferior to the anterior side of the tympanic perforation is luxated. Superiorly, starting from the chordal eminence, the tympanic membrane is slowly dislocated up to the malleus handle.

The posterior half of the tympanic membrane is elevated to expose the posterior quadrants of the tympanic cavity.
Fig. 4.39

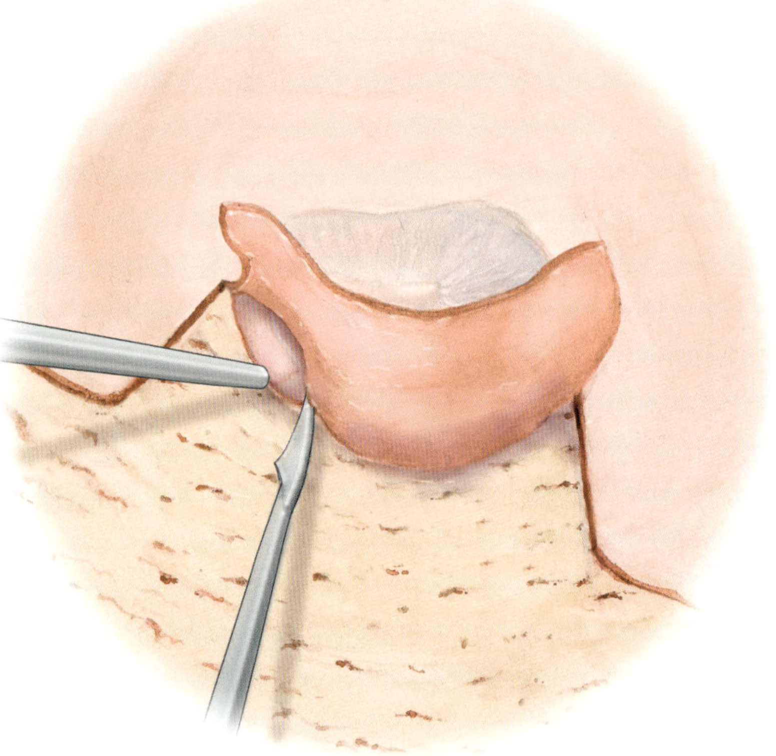

Fig. 4.38

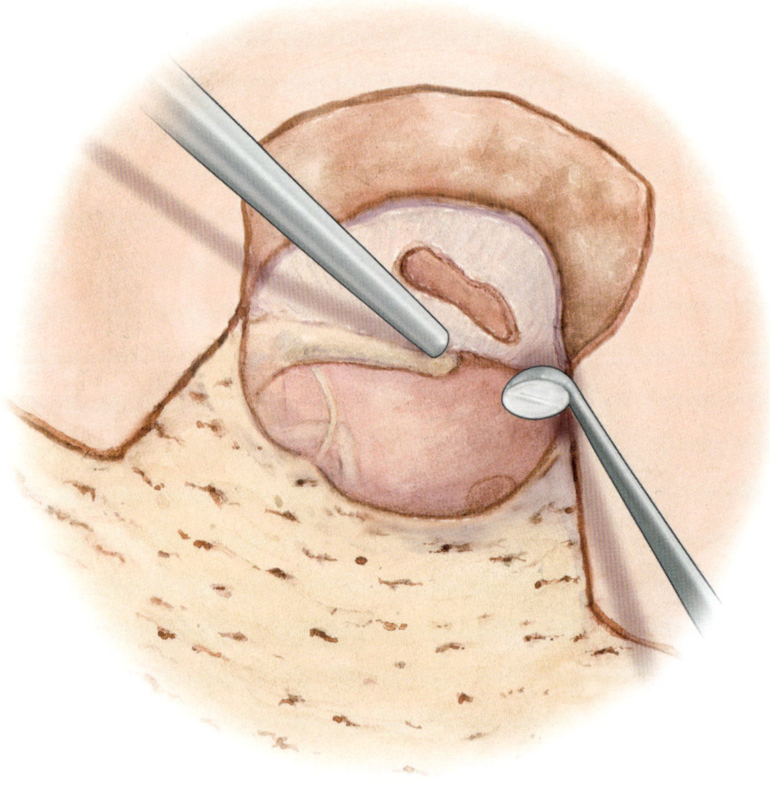

Fig. 4.39

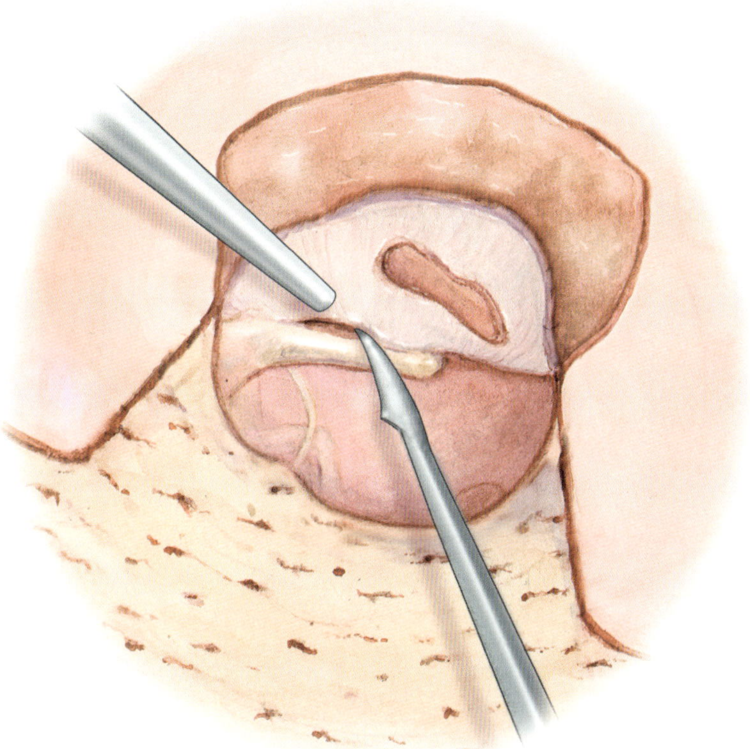

Fig. 4.40

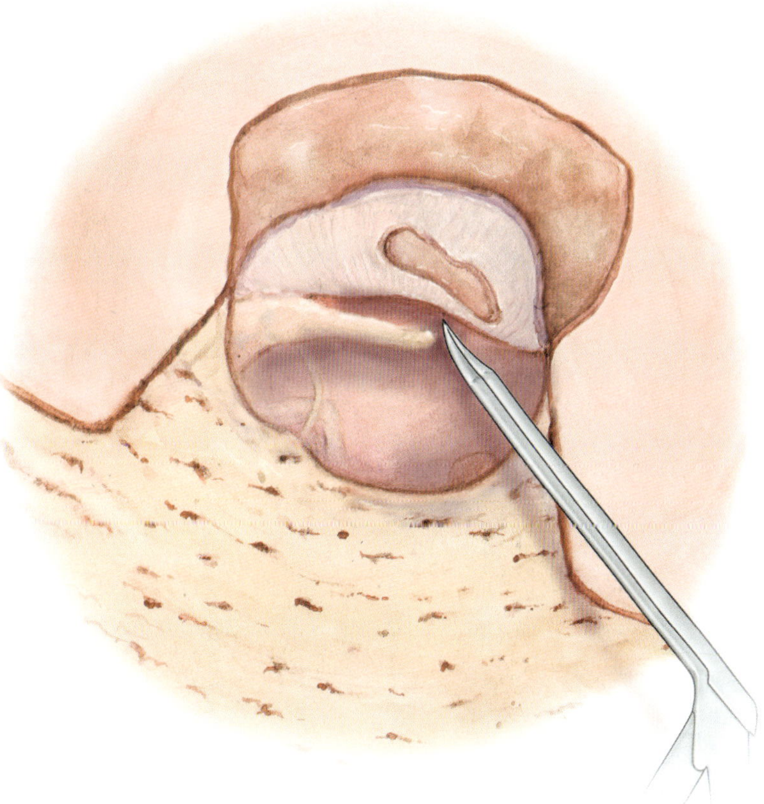

Fig. 4.41

Elevation of the Tympanic Membrane from the Malleus Handle

The epithelium on the malleus handle is elevated using a sickle knife, starting in the middle of the malleus handle where it is easier to detach. Longitudinal movements are required to prevent trauma to the ossicular chain and damage to the inner ear.

Fig. 4.40

Umbo Detachment

The umbo of the malleus handle is then detached using the same instrument or cut with microscissors. Finally, the malleus handle is cleared of any possible residual epithelium.

Ossicular chain mobility is checked using a needle and pulling the manubrium laterally (see Checking Ossicular Chain Mobility, p. 48).

Fig. 4.41

Tip: Residual epithelium pulls away easily. Fibrous tissue stays firmly attached and is difficult to remove. Do not forget to check the inferior side of the eardrum for epithelial remnants

Movements must be parallel to the axis of the malleus handle. If there is any doubt regarding the mobility of the ossicular chain, check the mobility of the round window. Place a drop of water on the round window; it helps to see moving reflections

Preparation of the Temporalis Fascia Graft

When the temporalis fascia is completely dry, it is carefully detached from the metallic sheet using a microdissector. The graft is shaped with blunt, curved scissors. It must be large enough to cover the entire perforation and ensure broad attachment to the malleus handle, bony annulus, and meatus posteriorly and inferiorly. After cutting, the graft is positioned using microforceps.

Fig. 4.42

Tip: The graft should be the same size and shape as a normal little finger nail.

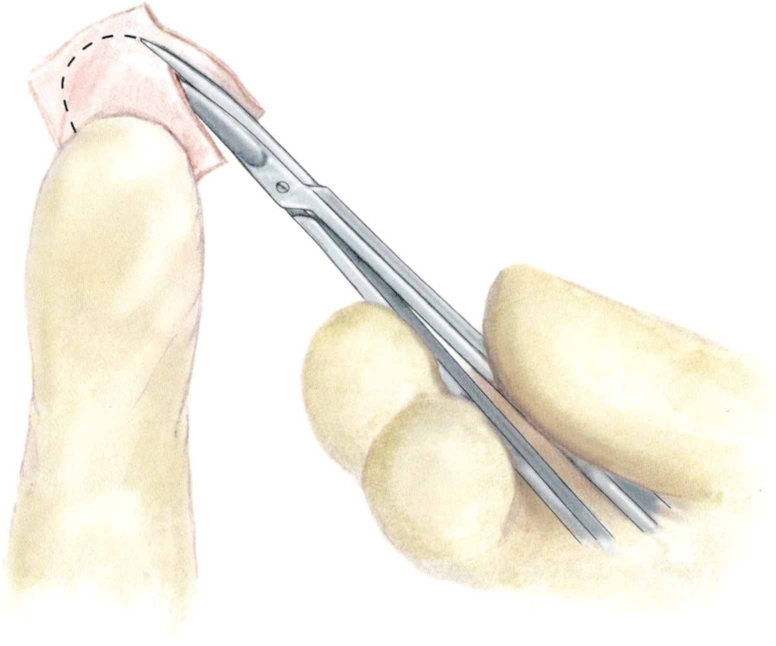

Fig. 4.42

Temporalis Fascia Graft Placement

The graft is slid between the malleus handle and the elevated tympanomeatal flap with microforceps and then under the anterior drum remnant. The position of the graft is adjusted to cover the denuded bone of the meatus inferiorly and posteriorly using a needle or spatula. The tympanomeatal flap is replaced. The position of the graft can be checked through the perforation and moved using a needle if necessary.

Fig. 4.43

Tip: Do not aspirate the graft and use small-diameter suction. Keep the graft dry until it is placed then add a few drops of water if necessary to soften it.

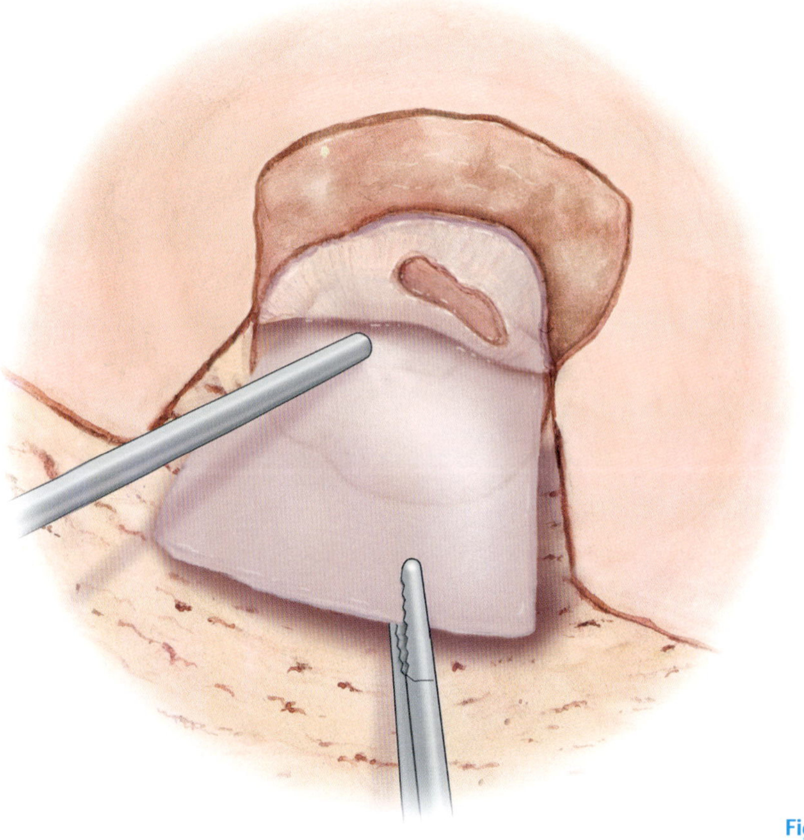

Fig. 4.43

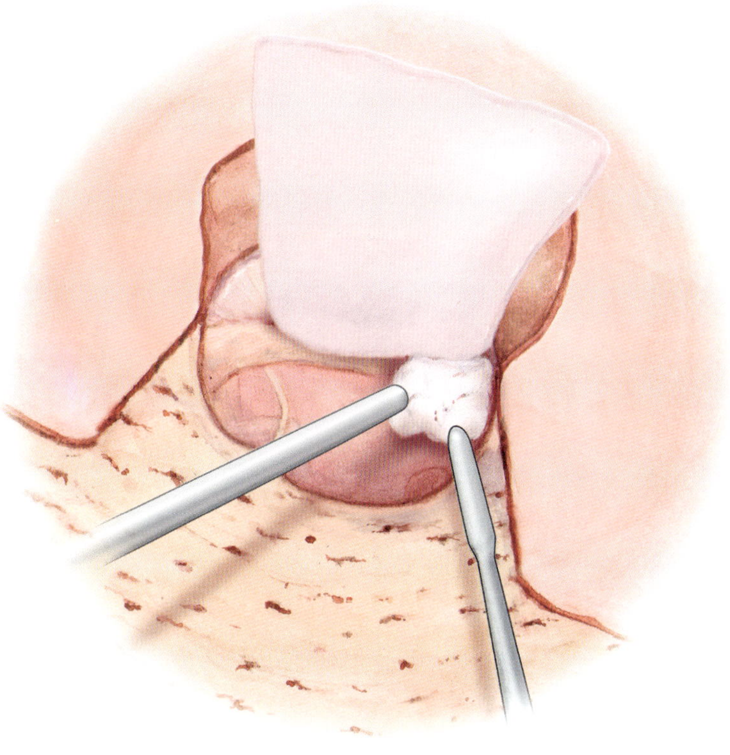

Fig. 4.44

Graft Stabilization

The graft and the tympanomeatal flap are re-elevated using a spatula. Hypotympanic and protympanic regions are filled with Spongostan (Johnson & Johnson Medical, Gargrave, Skipton, UK) soaked in physiological saline to support the graft anteriorly and inferiorly. Care is taken not to block the eustachian tube. The graft and the tympanomeatal flap are pulled down and stretched using small-diameter microsuction and a spatula, so as not to fold the skin, which may induce iatrogenic cholesteatoma. The tympanic reconstruction is fixed by applying fibrin glue to the surface of the perforation and by means of tympanomeatal flap incisions.

Fig. 4.44

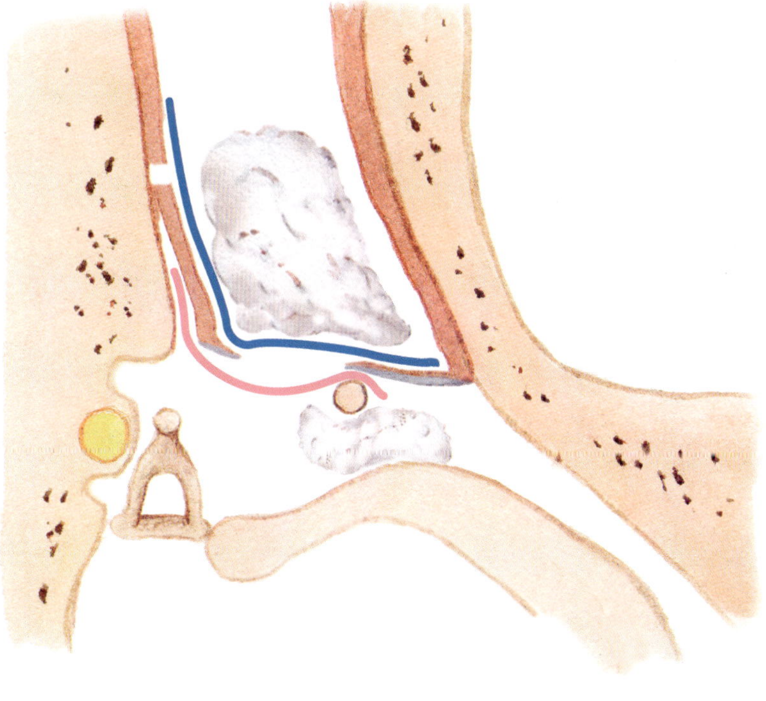

Fig. 4.45

Packing

A thin blue Silastic sheet is placed on the tympanic membrane and posterior wall. The canal is packed with Spongostan using a spatula and microsuction anteriorly first, then superiorly and inferiorly, taking care not yet to cover the posterior wall.

The Silastic sheet on the posterior wall is elevated, the mastoid retractor is removed, and the gauze string is cut at the level of the external canal and pulled out from the retroauricular side. The auricle is moved back into position after stretching the lateral meatal skin flap using anatomical forceps or a spatula. With a nasal speculum and spatula, the lateral meatal skin flap is replaced through the meatus. The Silastic sheet is pulled down and the packing is completed using large pieces of Spongostan.

Fig. 4.45

Tip: A blue Silastic sheet is easier to see than a transparent one when removing the packing.

Anterior Perforation

Meatal Skin Counterincision

The meatal skin counterincision is the same as that used for a posteroinferior perforation.

A circumferential incision of the laterally based meatal skin flap is made approximately 8 mm from the ear drum (see Incision Distance, p. 30).

Fig. 4.46

Optimal Exposure

The vascular strip is elevated with a strip of gauze and a self-retaining retractor is used to hold the musculoperiosteal and skin flaps in place.

Fig. 4.47

Excision of the Perforation Edge

The edge of the perforation is completely removed.

Fig. 4.48

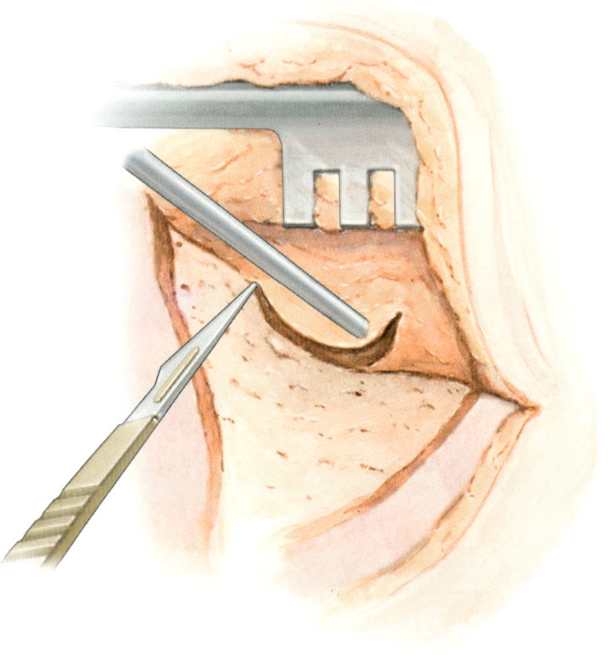

Fig. 4.46

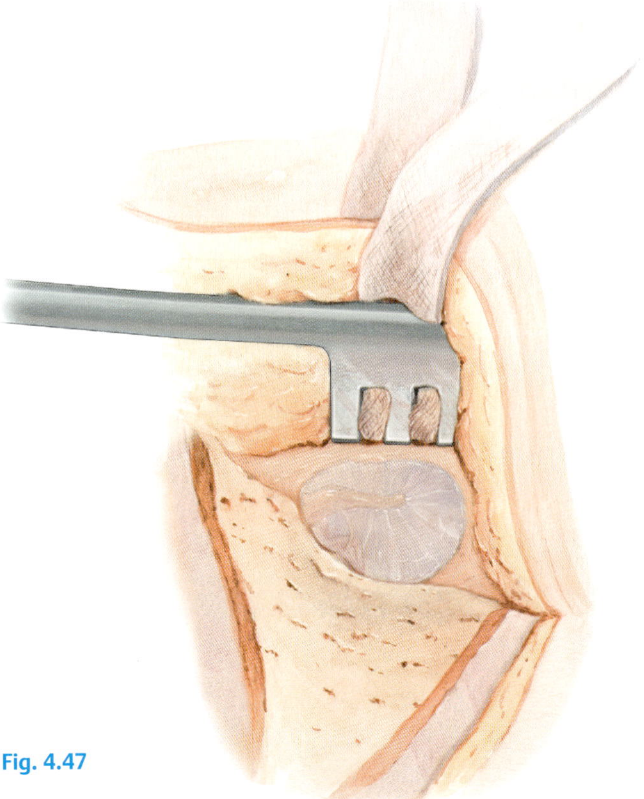

Fig. 4.47

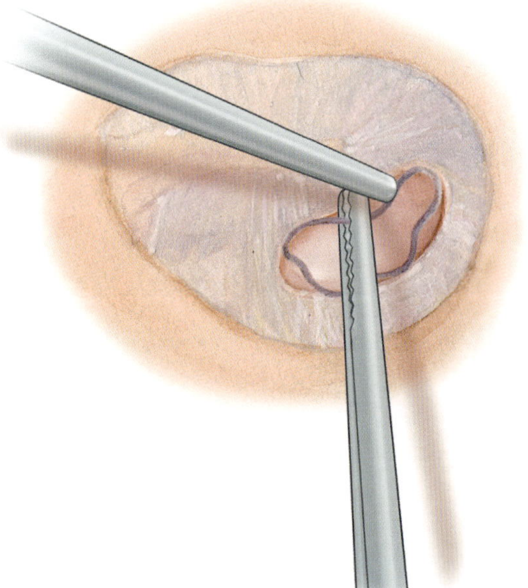

Fig. 4.48

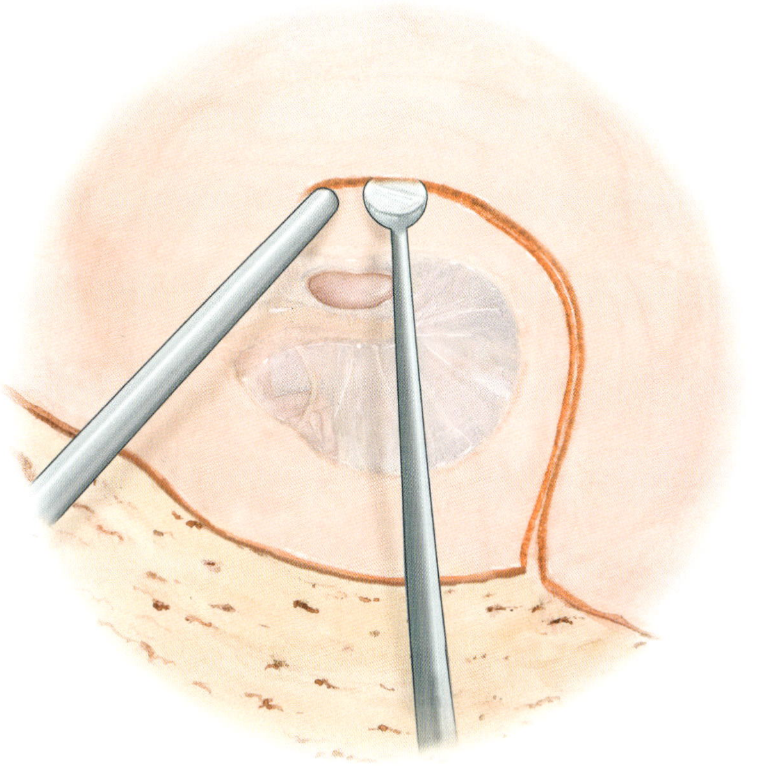

Fig. 4.49

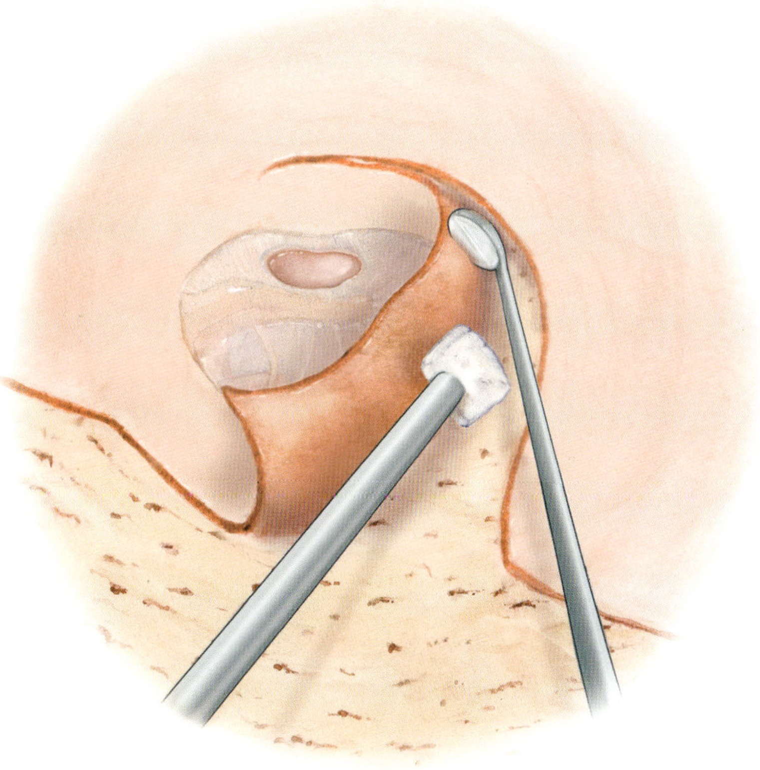

Fig. 4.50

Meatal Skin Incision

The circumferential skin incision is completed using a no. 11 scalpel blade or small round knife up to the inferior and anterior canal wall, localized approximately 8 mm from the eardrum.

Fig. 4.49

Meatal Skin Elevation

The posterior meatal skin is elevated toward the fibrous annulus with the round knife. Microsuction is performed with a small piece of Merocel or a cotton ball soaked in 1% lidocaine with 5 µg/mL epinephrine to protect the fragile skin and reduce bleeding.

Fig. 4.50

Tympanomeatal Flap Elevation

Using a needle or sickle knife, the fibrous annulus is dislocated out of the sulcus, beginning at the transition of the chordal eminence, paying particular attention to the chorda tympani. The middle ear mucosa must be incised to enter the middle ear cavity. When the opening is large enough, a flap knife or dissector-elevator is inserted and the fibrous annulus is luxated.

The posterior half of the tympanic membrane is elevated to expose the posterior quadrants of the tympanic cavity.

Tympanomeatal flap elevation is gradually continued along the inferior, then anterior canal wall to the superior level of the tympanic perforation. Elevation of the tympanic membrane from the malleus handle is required to complete the procedure. Tympanic membrane elevation is not needed above the chordal eminence.

The epithelium on the malleus handle is elevated using a sickle knife, starting in the middle, where it is easier to detach. Movements need to be longitudinal to reduce ossicular chain trauma and damage to the inner ear. The umbo is then detached using the same instrument or cut with microscissors. Finally, the malleus handle is cleared of any possible residual epithelium. Ossicular chain mobility is checked using a needle, pulling the manubrium laterally.

Fig. 4.51

Tip: Epithelial remnants are easy to remove. Fibrous tissue remnants are not.
In the case of anterior canal wall protrusion, the bony wall must be drilled (see Anterior Canal Wall Protrusion, p. 34).

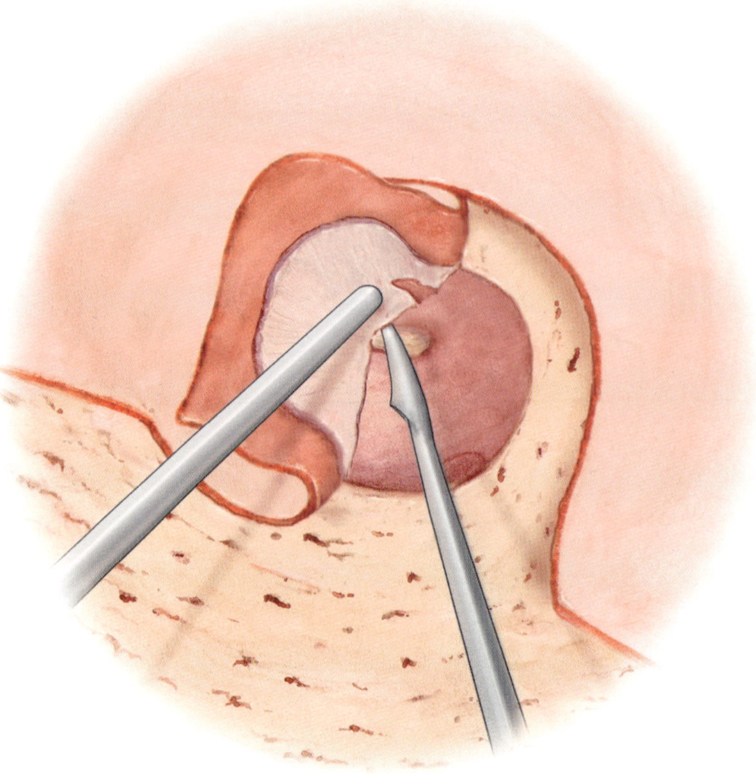

Fig. 4.51

Temporalis Fascia Graft Placement

The graft is slid between the malleus handle and the elevated tympanomeatal flap using microforceps up to the denuded bone of the anterior canal wall. The position of the graft is adjusted to cover the denuded bone of the anterior and inferior meatus and the malleus handle using a needle or spatula. The tympanomeatal flap is then replaced.

Fig. 4.52

Tip: Fold the tip of the graft. It allows easier placement on the anterior wall.

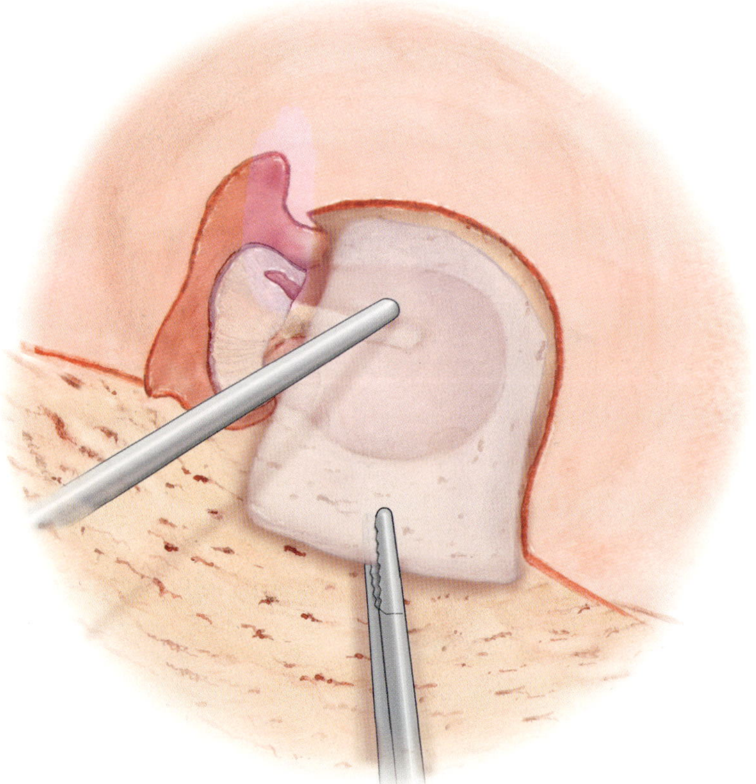

Fig. 4.52

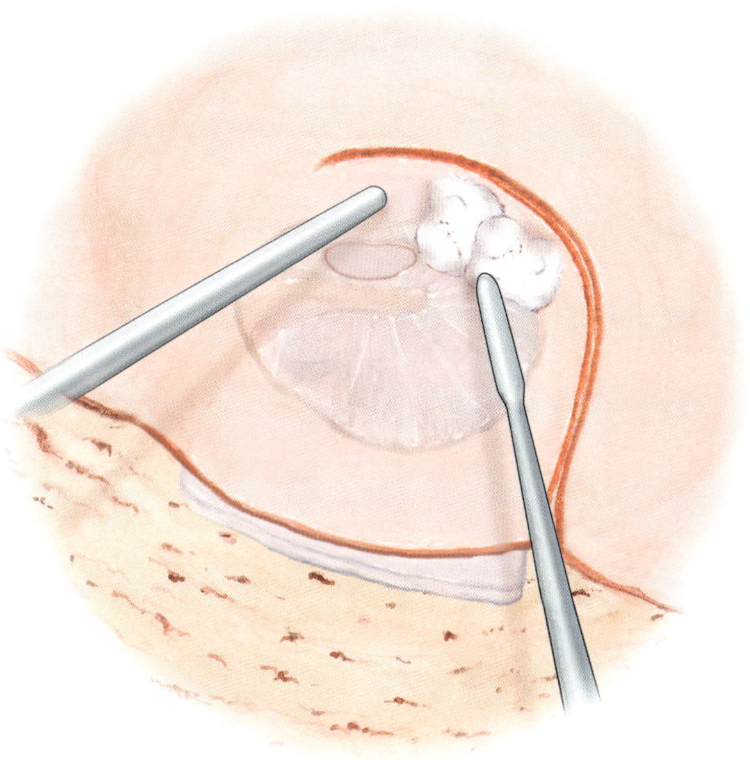

Fig. 4.53

Repositioning of the Tympanomeatal Flap

The graft and the tympanomeatal flap are pulled down and stretched using microsuction and a spatula, so as not to fold the skin, which may induce iatrogenic cholesteatoma. The tympanic reconstruction is fixed by applying fibrin glue to the surface of the perforation and by means of tympanomeatal flap incisions. Small pieces of Spongostan are pushed into the anterior angle.

Fig. 4.53

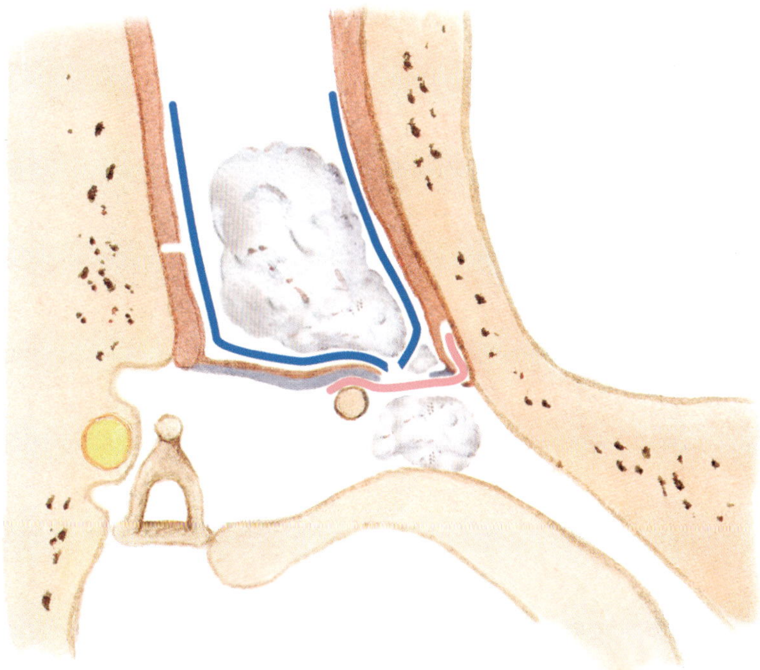

Fig. 4.54

Packing

A thin blue Silastic sheet is placed on the anterior wall, and another is positioned on the tympanic membrane and posterior wall and pushed onto the Spongostan to strictly restore the anterior angle. The canal is packed with Spongostan using a spatula and microsuction anteriorly first, then superiorly, and finally inferiorly, without covering the posterior wall. The Silastic sheet on the posterior wall is elevated, the mastoid retractor is removed, and the gauze string is cut at the level of the external canal and pulled out from the retroauricular side. The auricle is moved back into position after stretching the lateral meatal skin flap using anatomical forceps or a spatula. With a nasal speculum and spatula, the lateral meatal skin flap is replaced through the meatus. The Silastic sheet is pulled down and the packing is completed with large pieces of Spongostan.

Fig. 4.54

Total and Subtotal Perforation

Meatal Skin Counterincision

The meatal skin counterincision needs to be as close as possible to the annulus. It requires complete elevation of the posterior meatal skin between the two bony sutures.

A circumferential incision of the laterally based meatal skin flap is made at the level of the eardrum (see Incision Distance, p. 30). The vascular strip is elevated with a strip of gauze and a self-retaining retractor is used to hold the musculoperiosteal and skin flaps in place.

Fig. 4.55

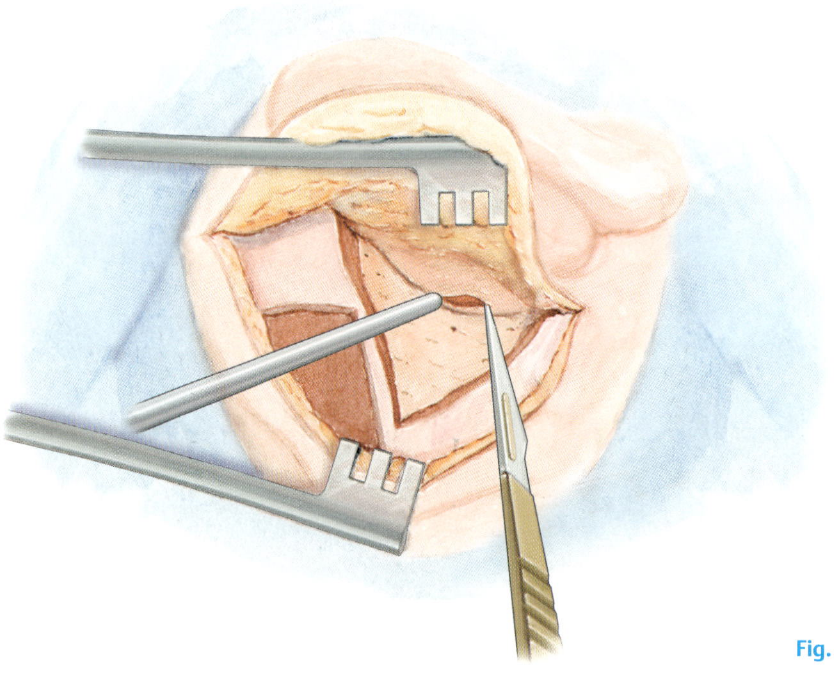

Fig. 4.55

Tip: The vascular strip needs to be as wide as possible. The end of the flap, protected by a sheet of Merocel because of its fragility, requires careful manipulation with small-diameter microsuction.

Anterior Meatal Skin Flap Incision

A circumferential skin incision, mostly blind, is made using a round knife or no. 11 scalpel blade just above the annulus, if possible.

Fig. 4.56

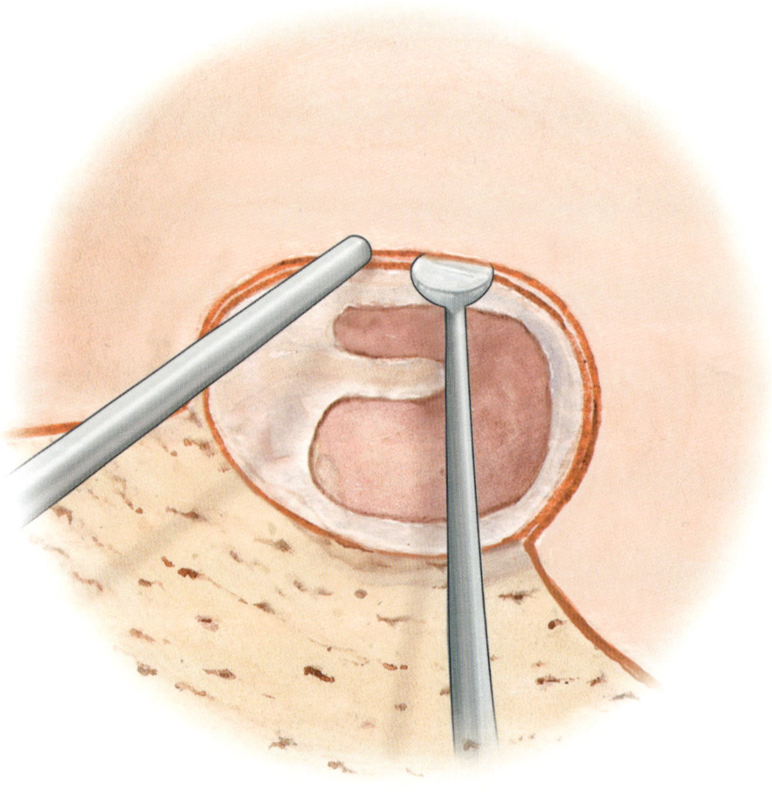

Fig. 4.56

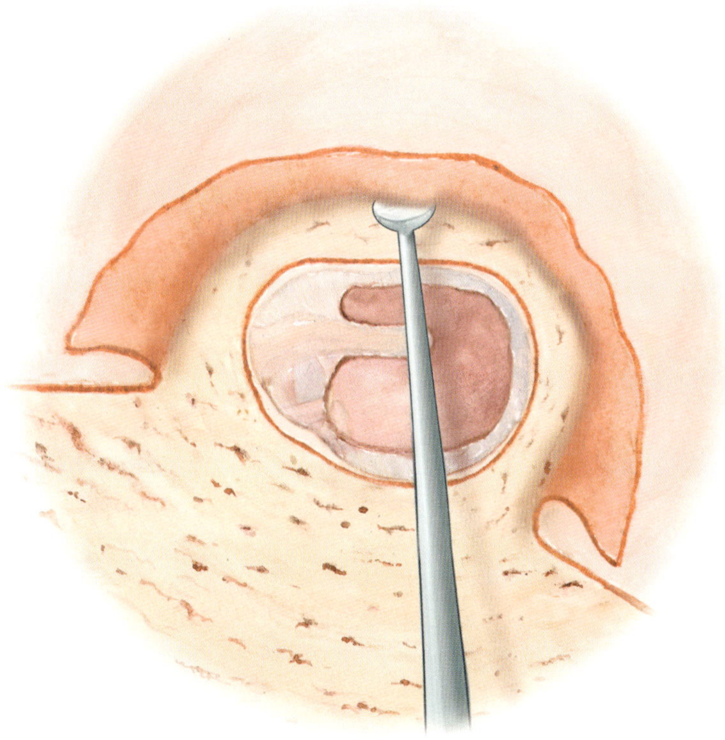

Fig. 4.57

Anterior Skin Flap Elevation

The meatal skin is first elevated from the bone above the annulus, along the circumferential incision, then pulled up gradually by 1 cm. The skin is folded back on itself and flattened onto the external canal.

Fig. 4.57

Tip: If the view of the anterior angle is not sufficient, it is necessary to drill the anterior bony canal with a small diamond burr. Care must be taken not to damage the elevated skin flap. Do not hesitate to elevate the anterior skin flap by 1 cm or more, as it improves visualization.

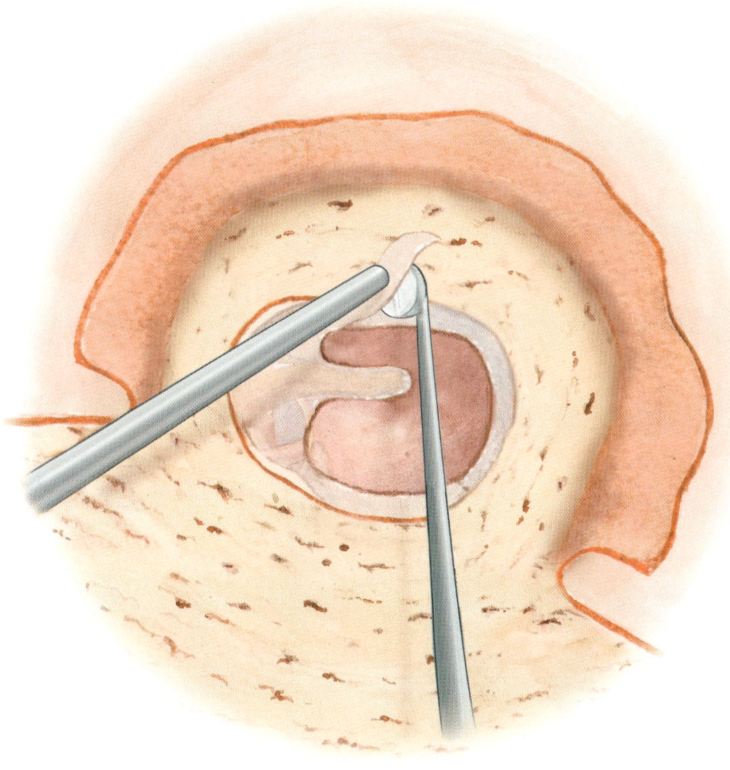

Fig. 4.58

Cleaning of the Tympanic Membrane

The residual keratinized squamous epithelium is removed from the tympanic membrane remnant, the annulus, and the malleus handle using microforceps, a round knife, or a small dissector-elevator. Cleaning must be meticulous and complete to avoid iatrogenic cholesteatoma.

Fig. 4.58

Excision of the Perforation Edge

The edge of the perforation is completely removed (see Excision of the Perforation Edge, p. 36).

Checking Ossicular Chain Mobility
Ossicular chain mobility is checked using a needle, pulling the manubrium laterally.

Fig. 4.59

Sometimes, the posterior tympanic membrane remnant blocks the view of the incudostapedial complex and this remnant must be elevated.

With a needle or sickle knife, the fibrous annulus is dislocated out of its sulcus, beginning at the chordal eminence transition, taking care not to touch the chorda tympani. The middle ear mucosa must be incised to enter the middle ear cavity. When the opening is large enough, a flap knife or dissector-elevator is inserted and the fibrous annulus is luxated.

The posterosuperior part of the tympanic membrane is elevated to expose the posterosuperior quadrant of the tympanic cavity.

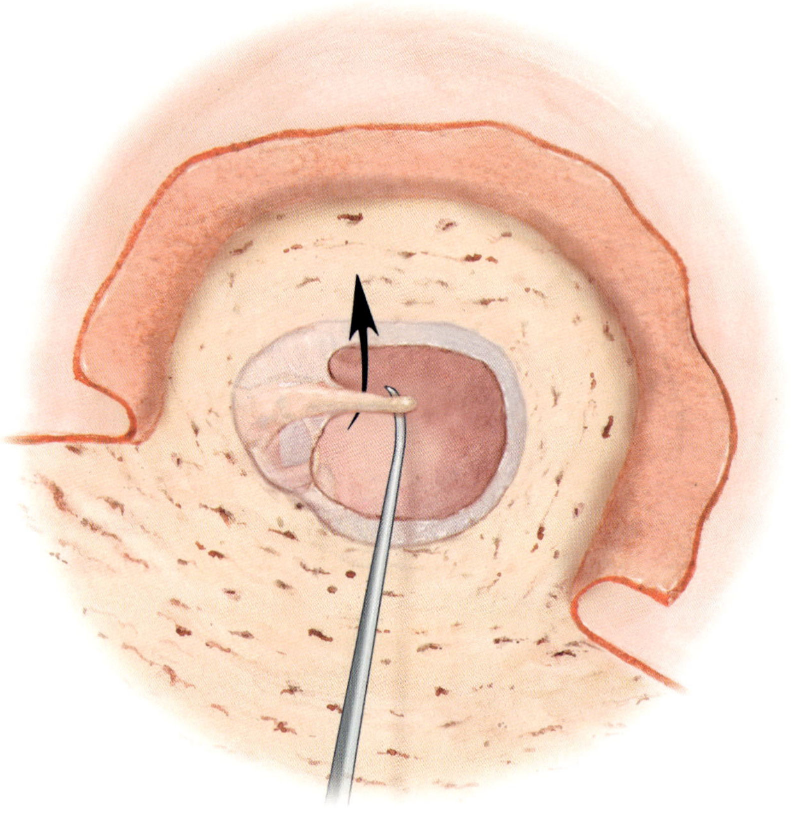

Fig. 4.59

Temporalis Fascia Graft Placement
When the temporalis fascia is completely dry, it is detached carefully from the Perkins mold using a microdissector or periosteal elevator. The graft is shaped using blunt curved scissors, respecting the mold shape. It must be large enough to cover the entire tympanic membrane surface, the bony annulus, and the meatus with a margin of at least 5 mm. After cutting, the graft is placed using microforceps.

The graft is slid onto the tympanic membrane remnant with microforceps. Using a needle or spatula, the position of the graft is adjusted to cover the denuded bone of the meatus with a minimum overlap of 5 mm. A mark is made on the graft with an electrocautery needle at the level of the superior half of the malleus handle.

Fig. 4.60

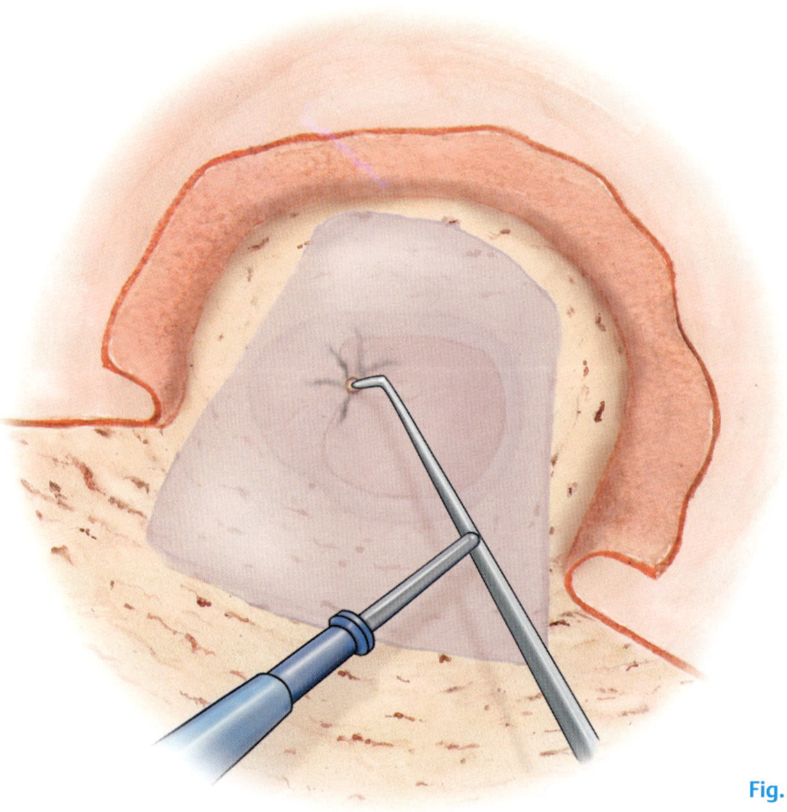

Fig. 4.60

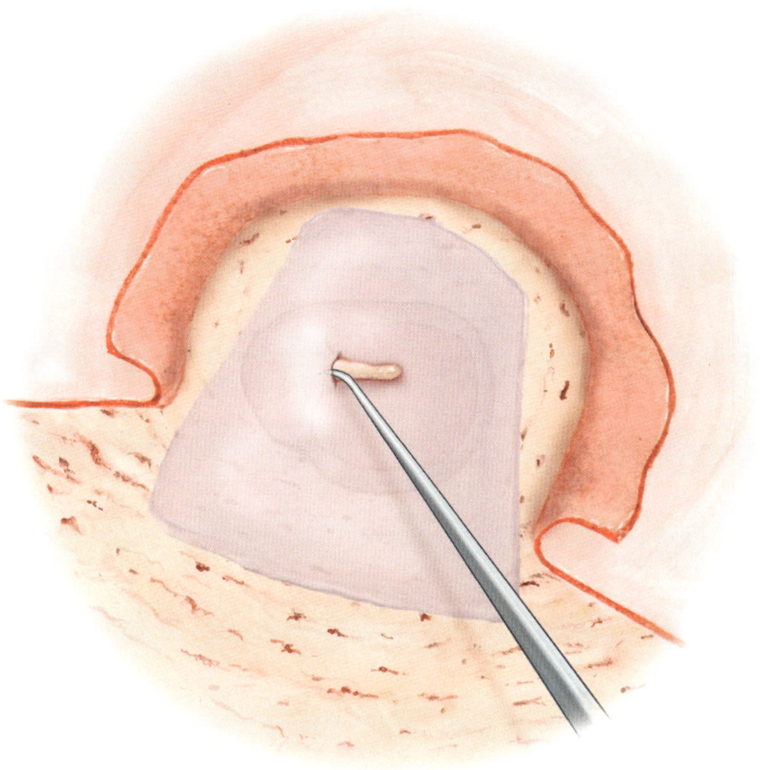

Fig. 4.61

Graft Button Hole

The graft is removed and placed on a wooden tongue depressor. A small buttonhole is cut using a no. 11 scalpel blade on the cauterized mark.

The graft is then replaced and the tip of the manubrium is passed through the buttonhole using microsuction and a needle.

The graft is positioned to cover the annulus and the denuded bone of the meatus with a minimum overlap of 5 mm all around to avoid blunting. The conical aspect of the tympanic membrane must be restored

Fig. 4.61

Tip: Try to keep the graft dry for this procedure.

Tip: When the graft is in place, it can be hydrated with a few drops of water.

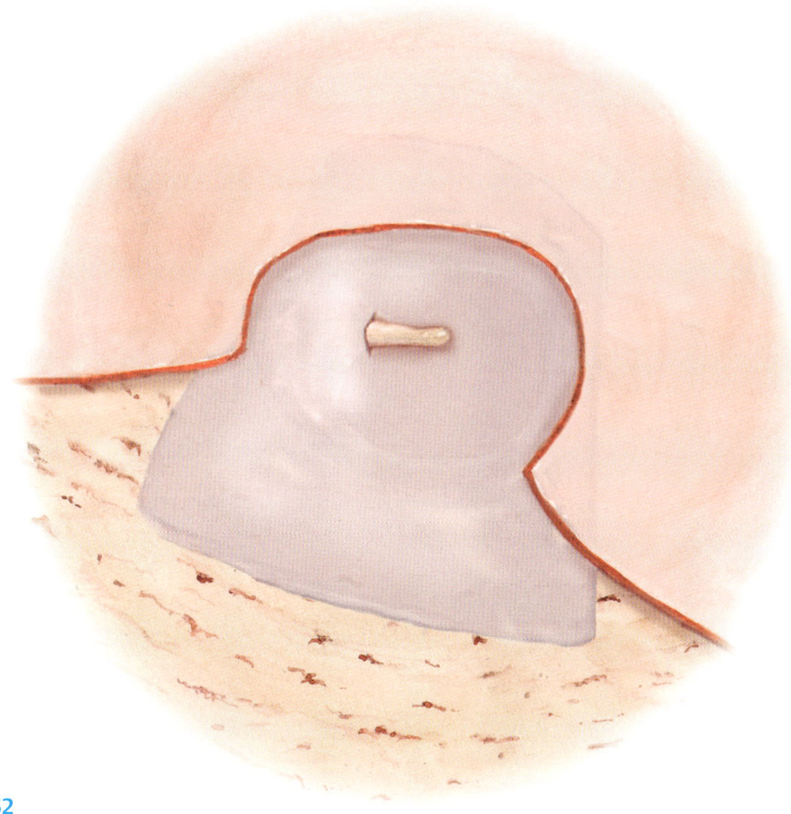

Fig. 4.62

Skin Flap Replacement

The anterior skin flap is returned and stretched using microsuction and a spatula, so as not to fold the skin, which may induce iatrogenic cholesteatoma. The tympanic reconstruction is fixed with fibrin glue.

Fig. 4.62

Tip: If the malleus handle is too retracted, do not make a buttonhole, but glue the graft onto the malleus handle. If the anterior meatal skin flap is too short, the uncovered bone must be covered with temporalis fascia. If the defect is too large, a free skin graft may be used.

Packing

Small pieces of Spongostan are pushed in the anterior wall.

A thin blue Silastic sheet is placed on the anterior wall. A second sheet is placed on the tympanic membrane and posterior wall, and pushed to strictly restore the anterior angle. The canal is packed with Spongostan using a spatula and microsuction anteriorly first, then superiorly, and finally inferiorly, taking care not to cover the posterior wall.

The Silastic sheet on the posterior wall is elevated, the mastoid retractor is removed, and the gauze string is cut at the level of the external canal and pulled out from the retroauricular side. The auricle is moved back into position after stretching the lateral meatal skin flap using anatomical forceps or a spatula. With a nasal speculum and spatula, the lateral meatal skin flap is replaced through the meatus. The Silastic sheet is pulled down and the packing is completed with large pieces of Spongostan.

Fig. 4.63

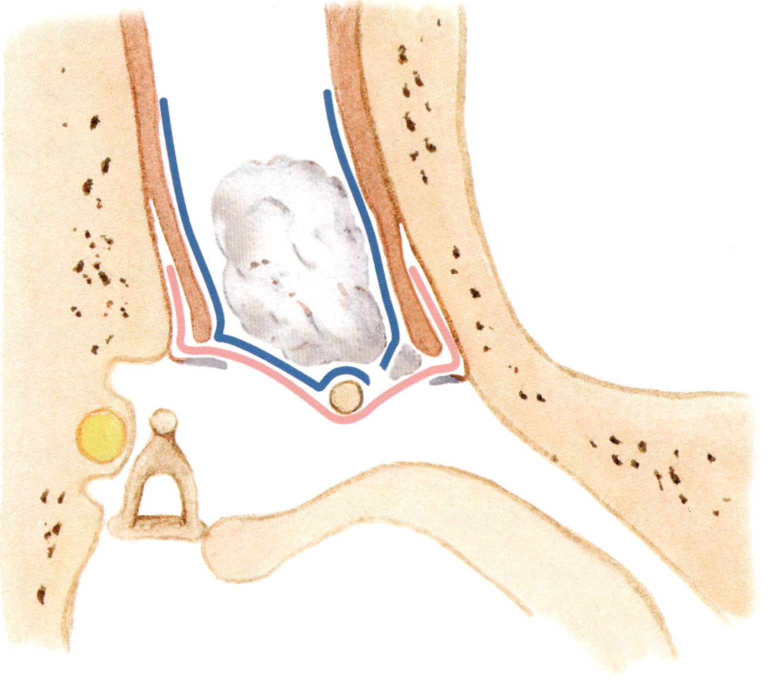

Fig. 4.63

Tip: To restore a perfect anterior angle, small Spongostan pieces can be inserted before placing the Silastic sheet. In the case of meatal skin flap defects and reconstructions with skin grafts or temporalis fascia, packing with Epifilm is performed.

Special Tympanoplasty Techniques and Problems

Tympanoplasty without Incision of the External Auditory Canal Skin

Indications for this technique are small or midsize perforations, not exceeding one-third of the tympanic membrane surface, located in the inferior or posterior quadrant. The patient's history may include prior tympanoplasty. The anatomy of the external auditory canal must allow total visibility of the perforation and the meatal skin must be of sufficient quality.

Tympanomeatal Skin Elevation

A classic retroauricular approach is initiated for temporalis fascia harvesting.

The posterior meatal skin is elevated to the sulcus with a periosteal elevator.

Using a dissector-elevator or lateral knife and microsuction protected with Merocel, cleavage is achieved between the epidermal and fibrous layers of the tympanic membrane. Epidermal debris on the tympanic membrane and the malleus handle is removed. The edge of the perforation is excised.
Fig. 4.64

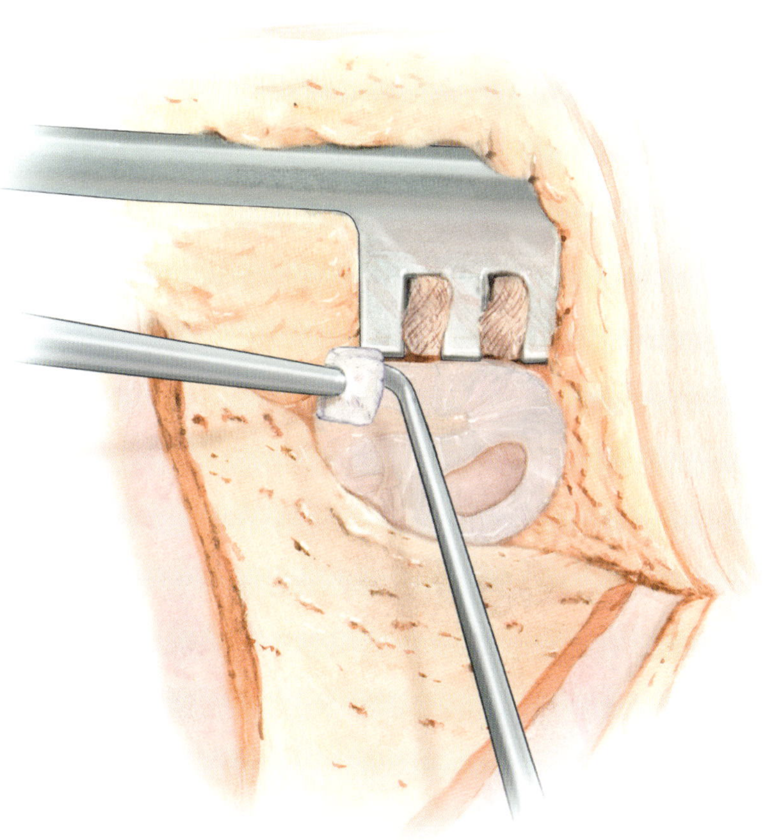

Fig. 4.64

Graft Placement

The temporalis fascia is then placed to cover the perforation and enough of the surface of the eardrum so as not to fall through.
Fig. 4.65

The ear is moved back into position.

There is quasi-spontaneous redraping of the tympanomeatal flap.

Packing is completed through the meatus with large pieces of Spongostan, using a nasal speculum, after depositing a small amount of fibrin glue onto the tympanic reconstruction.

Tip: Replacing the meatal skin is difficult. Packing large, dry pieces of Spongostan with a spatula helps. Be careful not to aspirate the graft with microsuction.

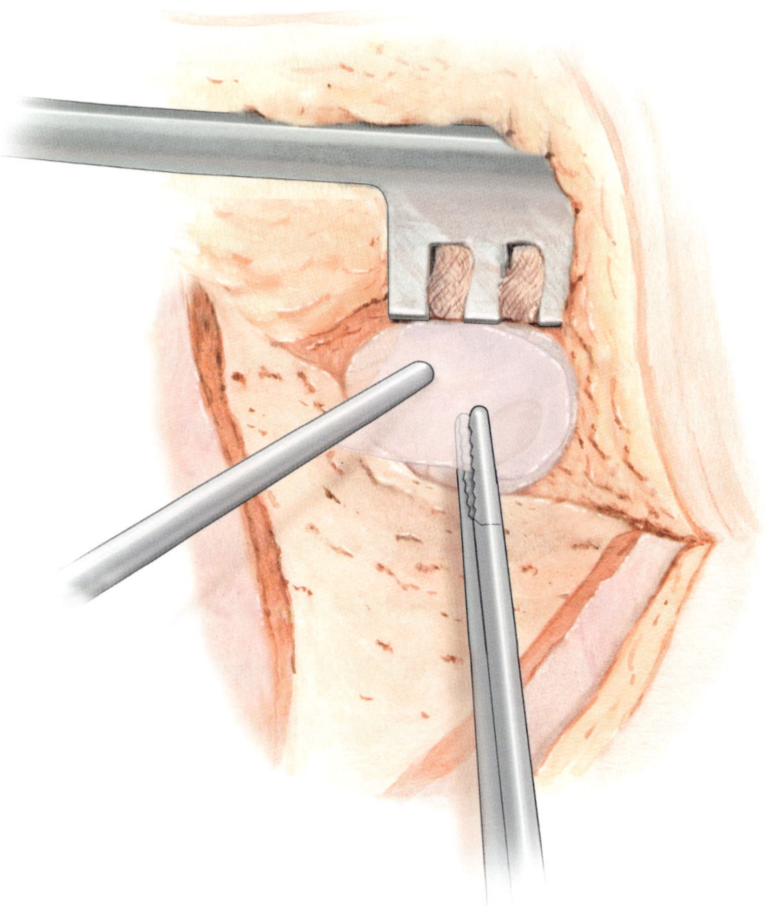

Fig. 4.65

Fatty Tissue Myringoplasty

This technique is used for small posterior or inferior perforations. We use it in association with conventional tympanoplasty of the contralateral ear.

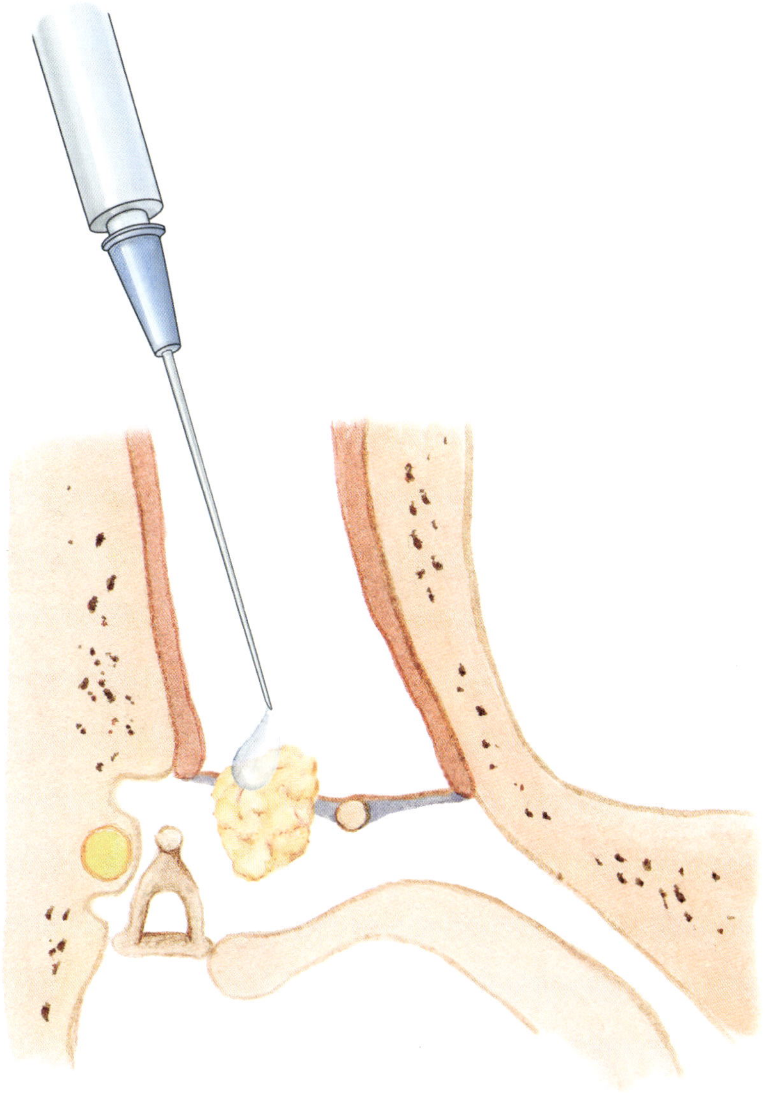

Fig. 4.66

Excision of the Perforation Edge
Using a sickle knife, the edge of the perforation is incised through all three layers of the eardrum. Numerous incisions are made around the circumference of the perforation. The edges are pushed toward the center and removed with microforceps (see Excision of the Perforation Edge, p. 42).

Fatty Tissue Placement
The fatty tissue from the ear lobe (see Fatty Tissue Graft, p. 26) or abdomen is dried of disinfectant solution and, with a needle or microforceps, used to plug the perforation, with 60% of its volume inside the middle ear and the rest outside. A small amount of fibrin glue and a sheet of Spongostan may be used to improve fixation.
Fig. 4.66

Transcanal Tympanoplasty

Autografts (temporalis fascia, perichondrium) or xenogenous grafts such as Tutopatch (Tutogen Medical Inc., Alachua, FL, USA) can be used for transcanal tympanoplasty.
Tutopatch contains bovine pericardium and is usually used as a prosthesis for the surgical repair of soft tissue deficiencies. This collagenous connective tissue combines mechanical strength, flexibility, and elasticity. Homograft dehydrated fascia (Tutoplast) can also be used.

Indications for this technique are small or midsize perforations, not exceeding one-third of the tympanic membrane surface, located in the inferior or posterior quadrant. The patient's history may include prior tympanoplasty.

The anatomy of the external auditory canal must allow total visibility of the perforation. Excision of the perforation edge is performed through a transcanal approach.

Meatal Skin Incision

The procedure starts with a Rosen incision, a curved incision from 12 o'clock to 6 o'clock, or to the anterior level of the perforation.
Fig. 4.67

Meatal Skin Elevation

The skin flap must be at least 6–8 mm long. It is elevated to the fibrous annulus, which is dislocated out of the sulcus.
Fig. 4.68

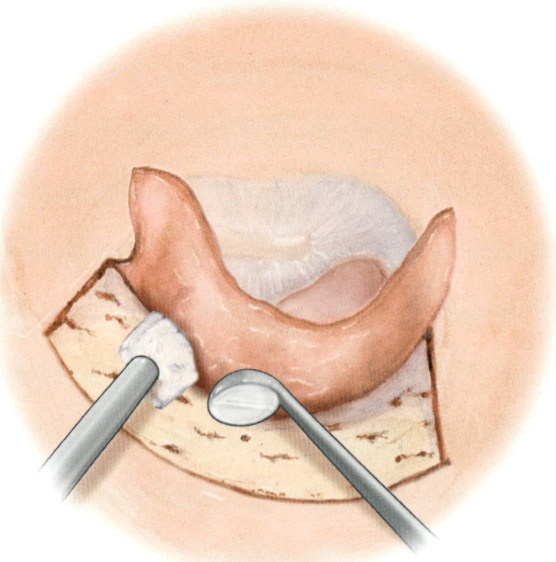

Fig. 4.67

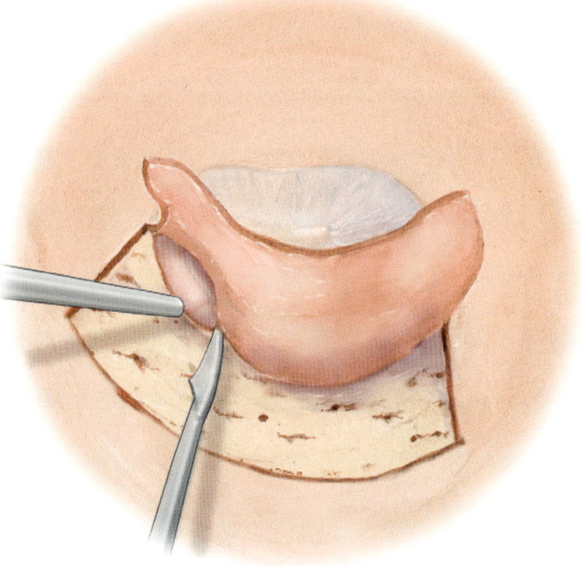

Fig. 4.68

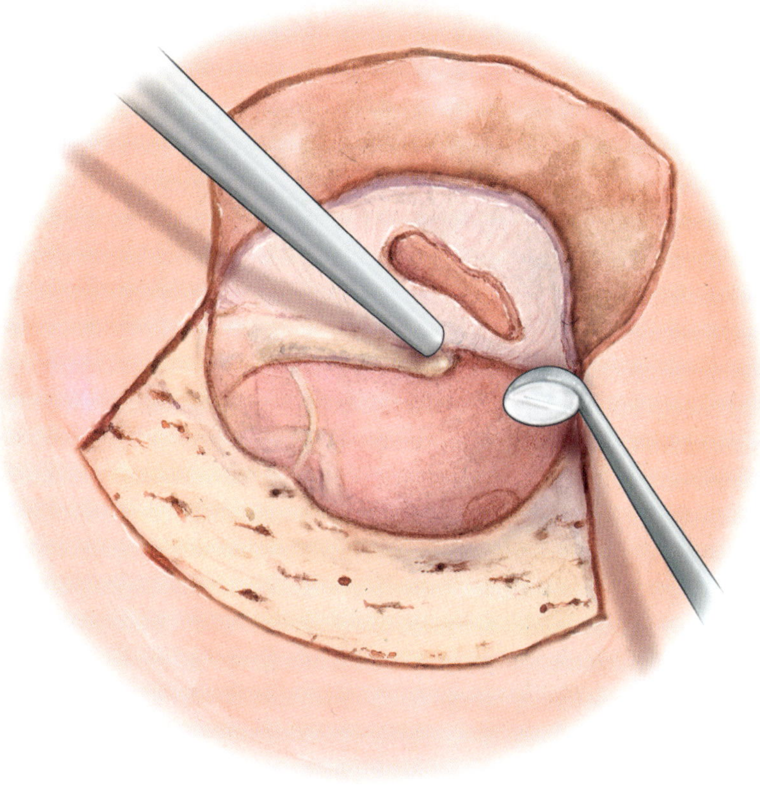

Fig. 4.69

Tympanomeatal Flap Elevation
Care is taken not to damage the chorda. Inferiorly, the annulus is luxated to the anterior level of the perforation. The mobility of the ossicular chain is checked.

Fig. 4.69

Elevation of the Tympanic Membrane from the Malleus Handle
The epithelium on the malleus handle is elevated using a sickle knife, starting in the middle of the malleus handle where it is easier to detach. Longitudinal movements are required to prevent trauma to the ossicular chain and damage to the inner ear.

Fig. 4.70

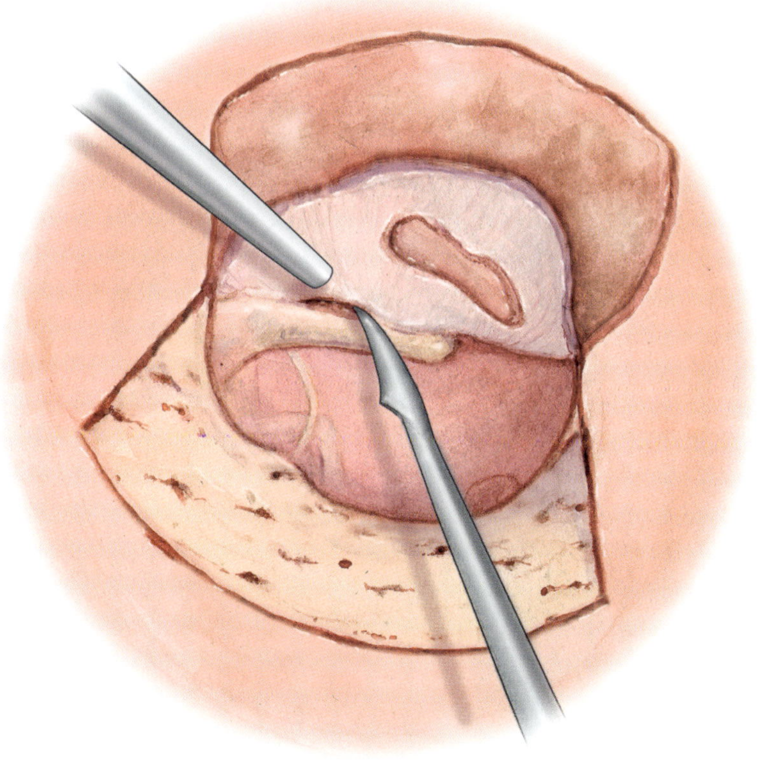

Fig. 4.70

Final Elevation

The tympanomeatal flap is finally elevated from the malleus handle.

Fig. 4.71

Graft Placement

The graft is shaped like a classic temporalis fascia graft as a 14-mm diameter Tutopatch disk or a 3 × 2 cm sheet.

The graft is placed over the malleus handle, the annulus, and the denuded bone.

Fig. 4.72

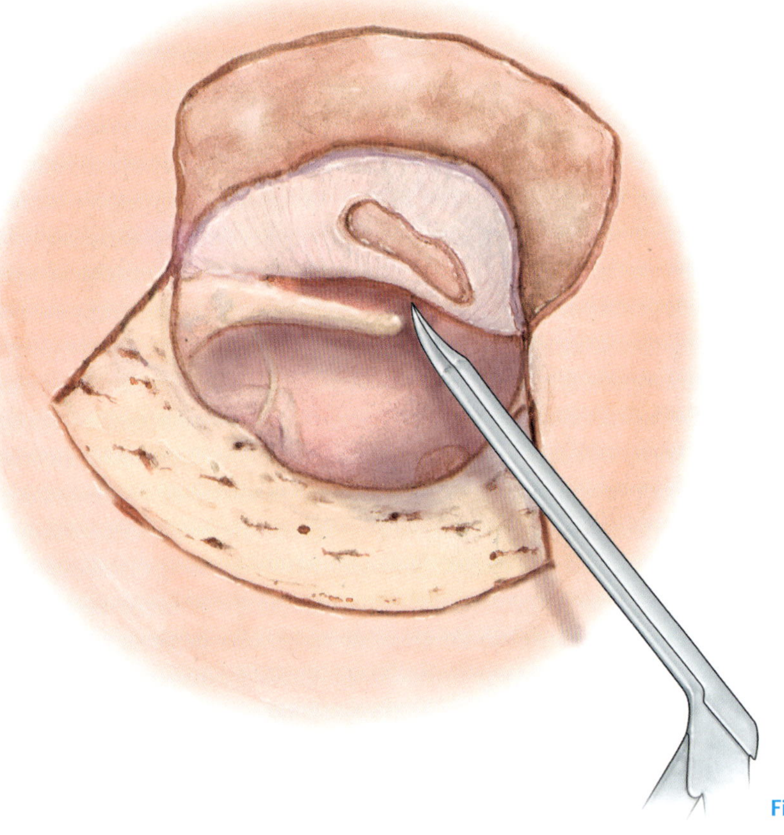

Fig. 4.71

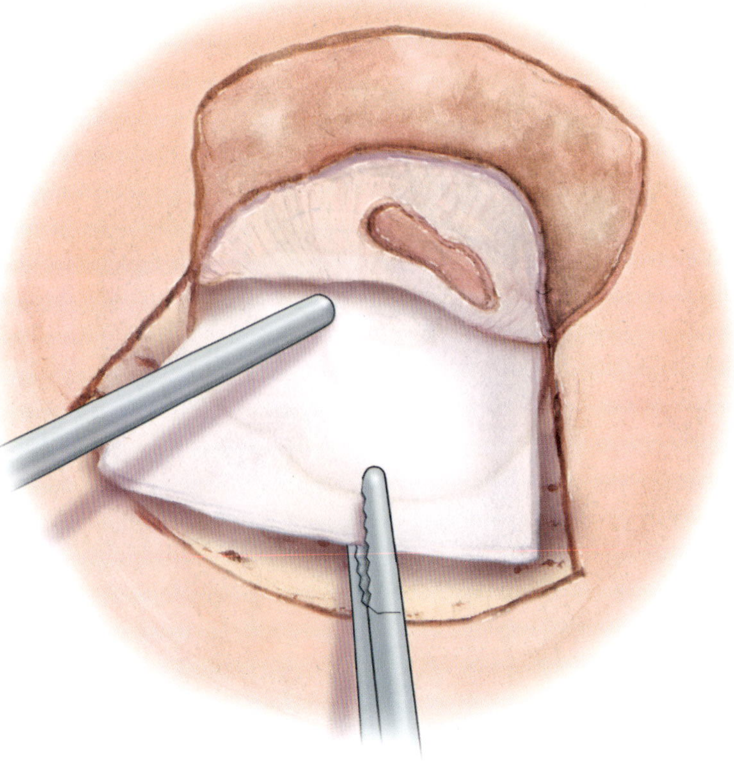

Fig. 4.72

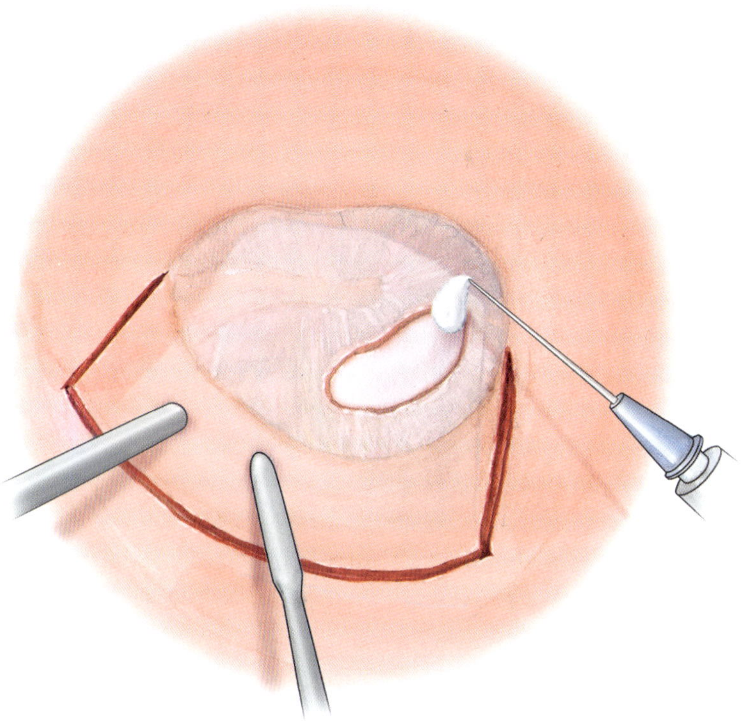

Fig. 4.73

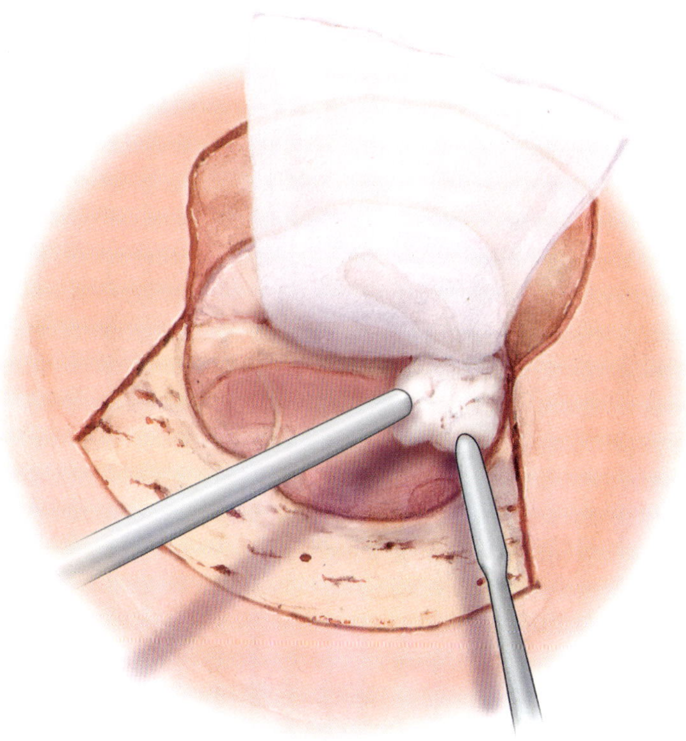

Fig. 4.74

Tympanomeatal Flap Replacement

For easier adjustment through the tympanic perforation when the tympanomeatal flap is replaced, the graft is positioned with the rough side facing up. The tympanic flap is fixed to the graft with fibrin glue.

Fig. 4.73

Graft Stabilization

The entire tympanic reconstruction is re-elevated and, using Spongostan, the graft is pushed upward into the hypotympanic area. Everything is then replaced and the external auditory canal is packed with Spongostan.

Fig. 4.74

Tutopatch can be used in exactly the same way as autografts and appears to produce the same anatomical and functional results without graft harvesting

Its texture, between that of temporalis fascia and perichondrium, is easy to handle, shape, and place.

There are several potential advantages to using Tutopatch, which include eliminating donor site morbidity, reducing operating time, and preserving native tissue for later use. It can also be successfully used in cases such as revision tympanoplasty, when standard tissue grafts are not available or are difficult to obtain.

Myringoplasty with a Hyaluronic Acid Patch (Epifilm)

We use this transcanal approach for small traumatic or residual perforations after grommets.

Excision of the Perforation Edge

Using a sickle knife, the edge of the perforation is incised through all three layers of the eardrum. Numerous incisions are made around the circumference of the perforation.

Fig. 4.75

Edge Removal

The edges are pushed toward the center using a needle or sickle knife, and removed with microforceps. Bleeding indirectly helps to close the perforation.

Fig. 4.76

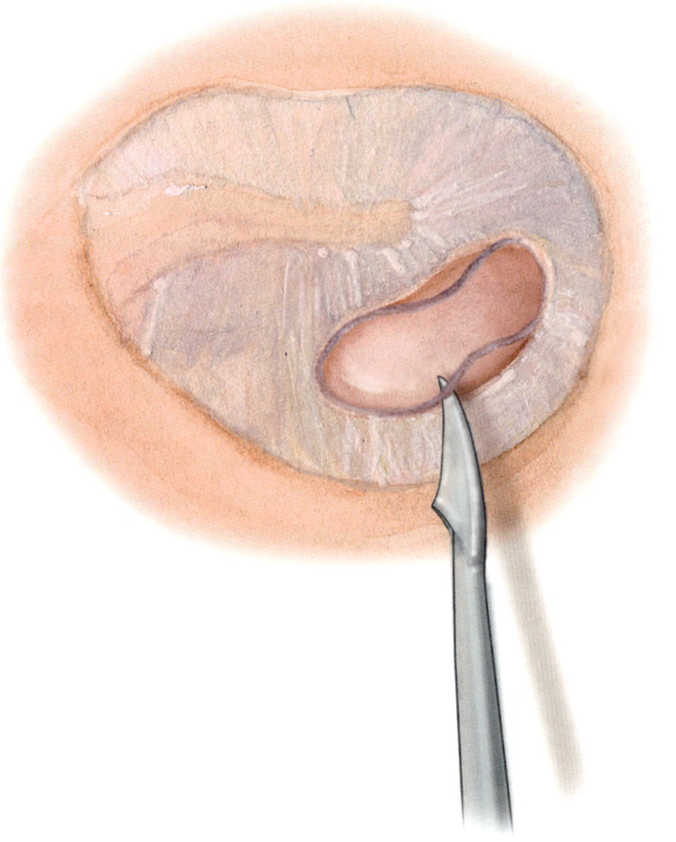

Fig. 4.75

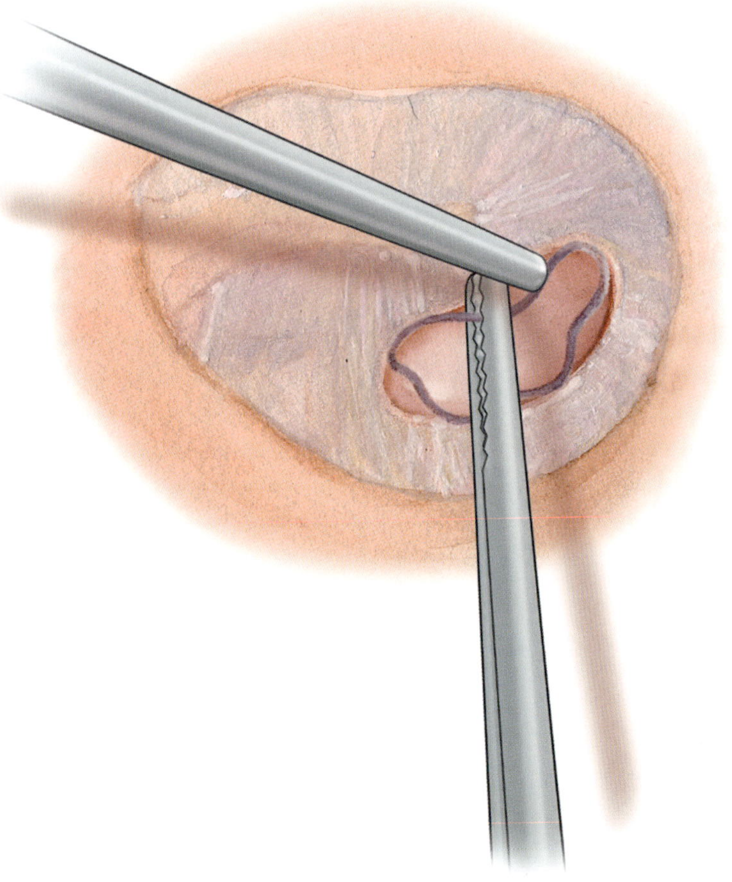

Fig. 4.76

Epifilm Placement

A round sheet of Epifilm is placed over the entire tympanic membrane without touching the meatus to avoid rapid migration.
Fig. 4.77

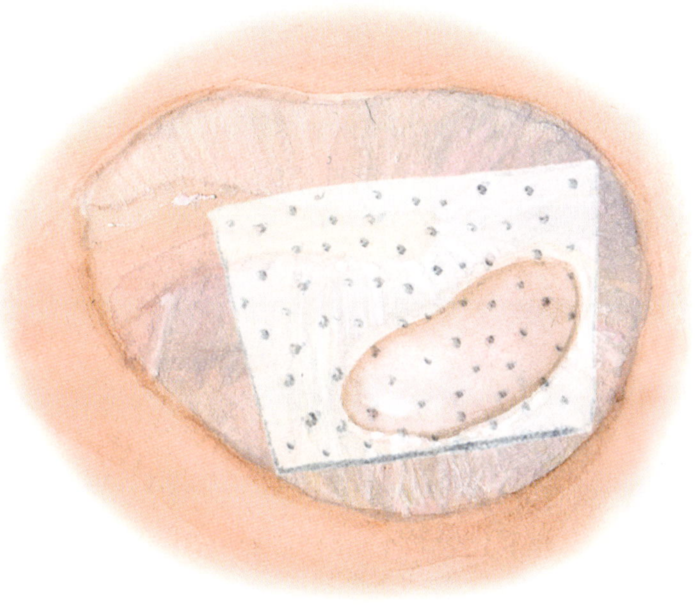

Fig. 4.77

Tympanosclerosis and Tympanoplasty

Tympanosclerotic plaques that touch the edge of the perforation, fix the ossicles, or obstruct the middle ear cavity should be removed.

Tip: Tympanosclerotic plaques of the anterior quadrant should be preserved, since they provide excellent support for overlay grafts.

Thickened Tympanomeatal Flap and Chronic Skin Inflammation

Chronic inflammatory tissue on the inferior side of the tympanomeatal flap must be partially excised to reduce the thickness of the flap. Chronic inflammation of the skin or everted mucosa (migration of the middle ear mucosa to the epidermic surface of the tympanic membrane and external auditory canal via the perforation) should be totally removed to guarantee good epithelialization.

Reconstruction of large meatal skin defects requires a free skin graft. Small defects can be reconstructed with fascia or perichondrium.

Tip: Bone defects should always be covered with a graft. Use of Epifilm facilitates healing.

Epithelialization of the Medial Side of the Tympanic Membrane and Middle Ear Extension

Limited skin extension on the medial side of the eardrum is removed using a small round knife to scratch the medial aspect of the tympanic membrane. In some cases, as a precaution, the tympanic membrane is also removed. Limited middle ear cavity extension should always be removed, except if there is round or oval window involvement, which requires second-stage surgery and the placement of a Silastic sheet in the middle ear. Cholesteatoma surgery is necessary if there is extensive cavity involvement.

Cartilage Tympanoplasty

Tragal cartilage, with or without perichondrium, or conchal cartilage is used for the treatment of atelectasis and retraction pockets and in revision surgery. The cartilage is placed to reinforce the pathological quadrants or the entire tympanic membrane. It can be used in one piece or many pieces can be set up in a palisade.

Total Cartilage Tympanoplasty

Cartilage Preparation

Refined tragal cartilage without perichondrium is shaped to the size of the tympanic membrane. The graft is slid onto the tympanic membrane remnant with microforceps, as in total tympanoplasty. A mark is made on the graft with an electrocautery needle at the level of the malleus handle.

A notch is made on a wooden tongue depressor using a no. 11 scalpel blade or lateral knife to allow insertion of the malleus handle.

Fig. 4.78

Tip: If the malleus is retracted, palisade cartilage tympanoplasty should be performed.

Cartilage Graft Placement

The cartilage graft is positioned overlying the residual tympanic membrane and underlying the malleus handle.

The cartilage is finally covered with temporalis fascia or perichondrium positioned on the cartilage and the denuded bone of the meatus with a minimum overlap of 5 mm.

Fig. 4.79

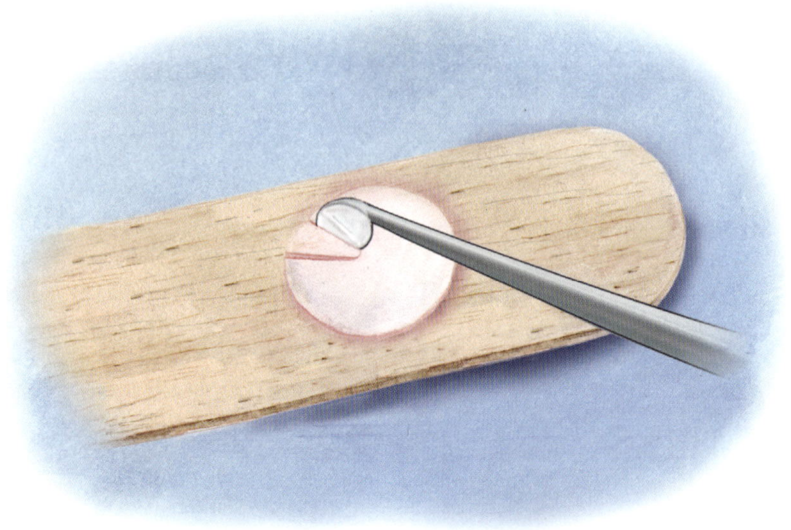

Fig. 4.78

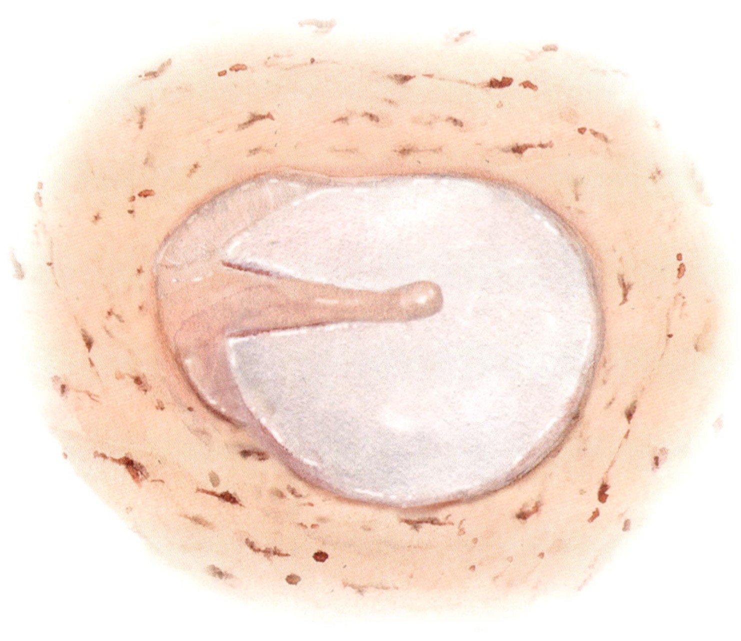

Fig. 4.79

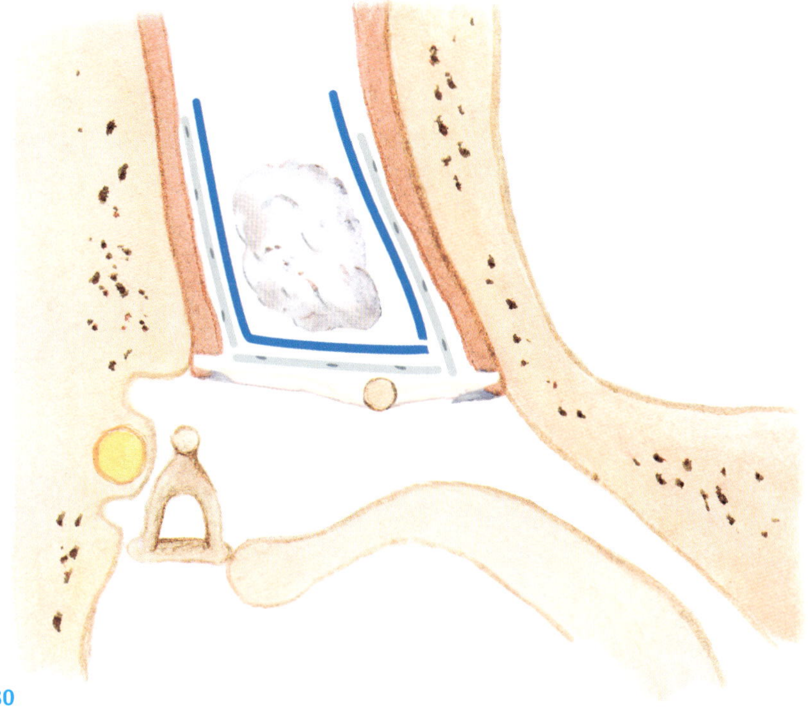

Fig. 4.80

The anterior skin flap is replaced and stretched using microsuction and a spatula, so as not to fold the skin, which may create iatrogenic cholesteatoma. The tympanic reconstruction is fixed with fibrin glue

Cartilage Tympanoplasty Packing

Packing is performed with Epifilm and Spongostan

Fig. 4.80

.

Posterior Cartilage Tympanoplasty

Cartilage–Perichondrium Graft Placement

When tragal cartilage is used, the perichondrium is kept attached to the cartilage.

When a tragal–perichondrium graft is used for recurrent perforation or retraction pocket, the cartilage covered with perichondrium covers the pathological quadrants and the perichondrium flap is placed on the posterior bony canal.

Fig. 4.81

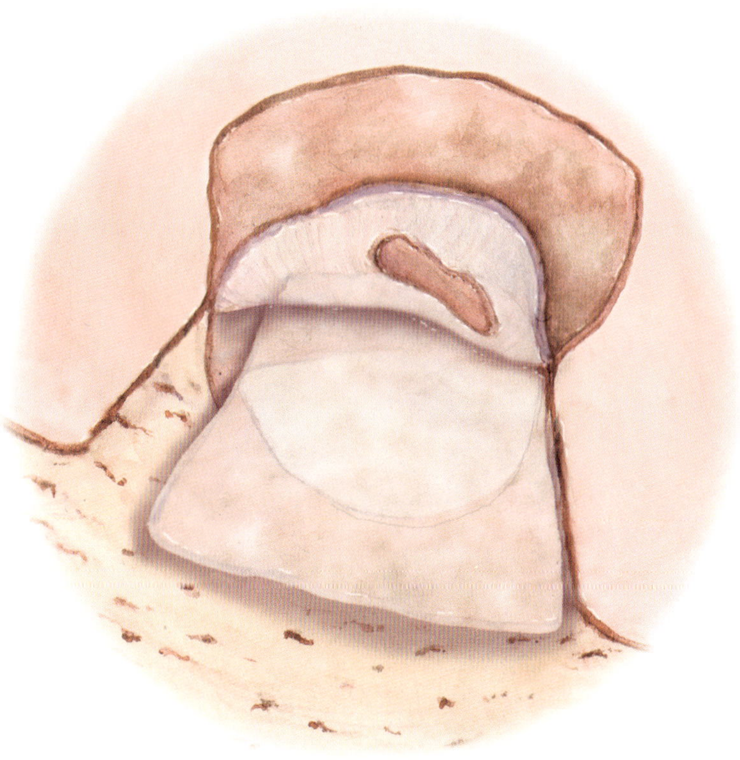

Fig. 4.81

Palisade Cartilage Tympanoplasty

Cartilage Chips Placement

Chips of tragal or conchal cartilage (see Graft Preparation, p. 24) are positioned like a puzzle to reconstruct or reinforce the tympanic membrane.

This is an excellent way of preserving the three-dimensional anatomy of the eardrum. Cartilage chips are fixed with fibrin glue and covered with a temporalis fascia or perichondrial graft.

Fig. 4.82

Tip: We prefer to use the palisade technique because the tympanic reconstruction can be adapted to anatomical constraints (retraction of the malleus handle, associated bony wall defects). Using small chips of cartilage allows greater flexibility in terms of cartilage shape, which is sometimes difficult to control or use for reconstruction purposes.

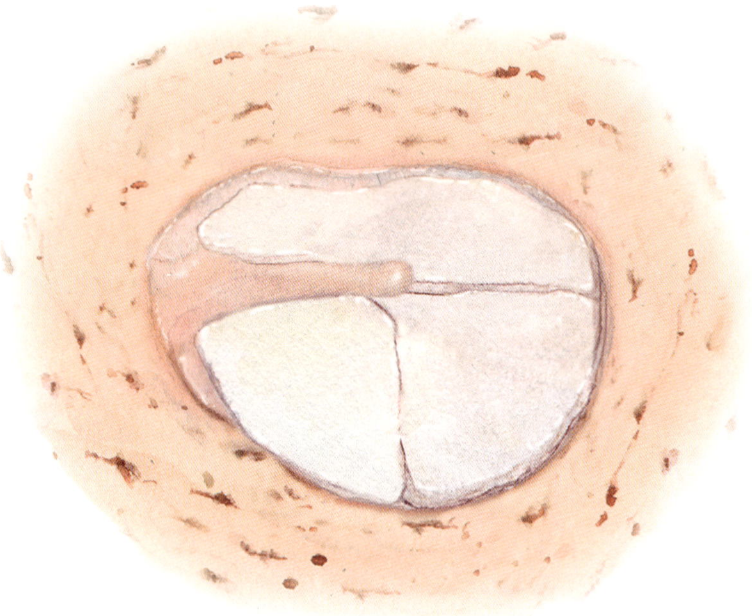

Fig. 4.82

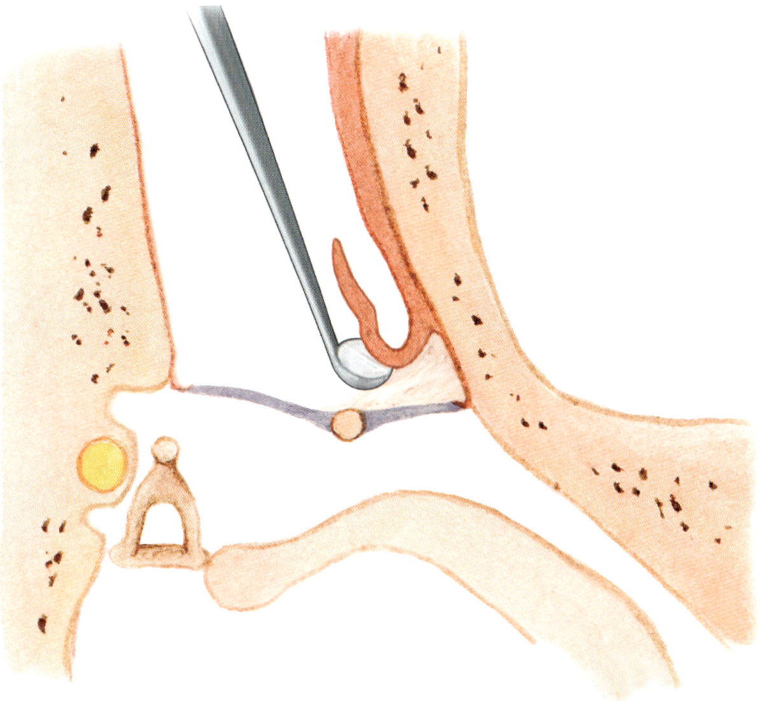

Fig. 4.83

Lateralization and Blunting

Elevation of the Tympanomeatal Flap Epidermis

The meatal skin counterincision needs to be as close as possible to the annulus.

Tympanic Skin Elevation

In cases of blunting, using a microdissector or lateral knife and protected microsuction, cleavage is achieved between the epidermal and fibrous layers of the tympanic membrane, and the epidermal layer is elevated to the anterior wall a few millimeters above the blunting.

Fig. 4.83

Fibrous Tissue Cleaning

The fibrous layer is cleaned of healing tissue to restore the anterior angle of the annulus.

Fig. 4.84

For lateralization of a healthy tympanic membrane, the three layers of the eardrum are elevated. If the annulus is absent, a new sulcus is created using a small diamond burr.

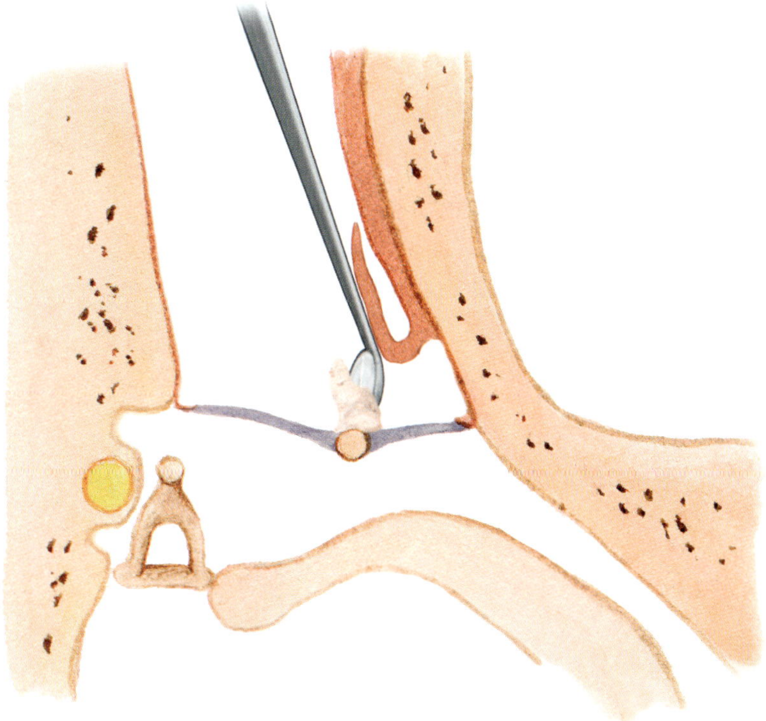

Fig. 4.84

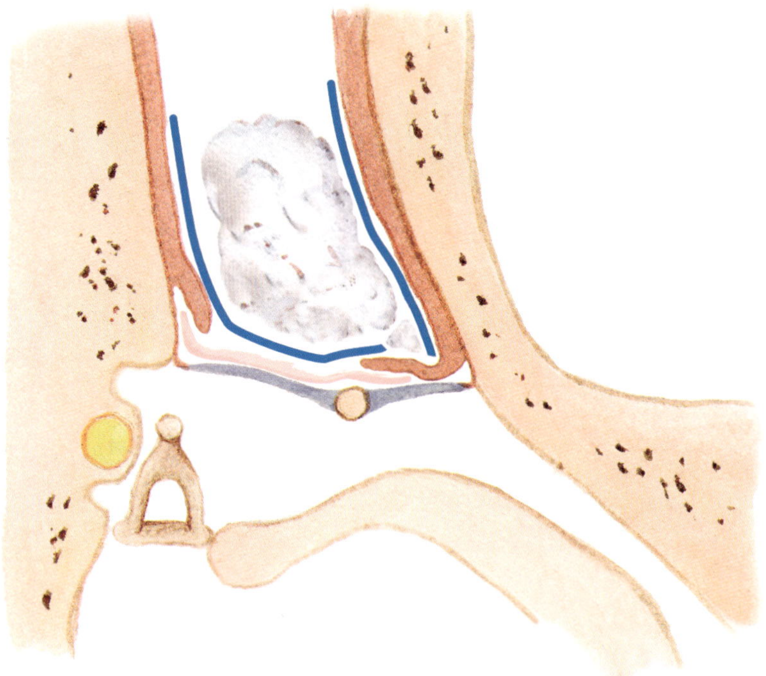

Fig. 4.85

Repositioning of the Tympanomeatal Flap

Temporalis fascia or a perichondrial graft can be used for tympanic reconstruction. In the case of blunting, the graft is positioned to cover the denuded bone of the posterior meatus and the surface of the fibrous tympanic layer, which will not be covered by the tympanomeatal flap. For lateralization, the tympanic membrane defect is reconstructed using a classic perforation technique, but the graft must be medial to the malleus handle if the malleus is present.

The tympanomeatal skin flap is replaced and stretched using microsuction and a spatula. The anterior angle is rigorously reconstructed. The tympanic reconstruction is fixed with fibrin glue.

A thin blue Silastic sheet is placed on the anterior wall, and another is used to cover the tympanic membrane and posterior wall, and is pushed to strictly restore the anterior angle. The canal is packed anteriorly with small sheets of Spongostan. The rest of the packing is done according to the classic procedure. Fig. 4.85

Skin and Musculoperiosteal Flap Closure

Musculoperiosteal flap and subcutaneous suture is performed using 3/0 Vicryl (Johnson & Johnson Medical). In adults, the skin is closed with stitches. In children the skin is glued or secured with Steri-Strips (3M, St. Paul, Minnesota, USA).

5

Management of Ossicular Abnormalities

5__Management of Ossicular Abnormalities

Tympanoplasty Classification

Type 1 Tympanoplasty

Any procedure of the tympanic cavity or middle ear with the conservation of an intact chain and tympanic membrane reconstruction.
Fig. 5.1

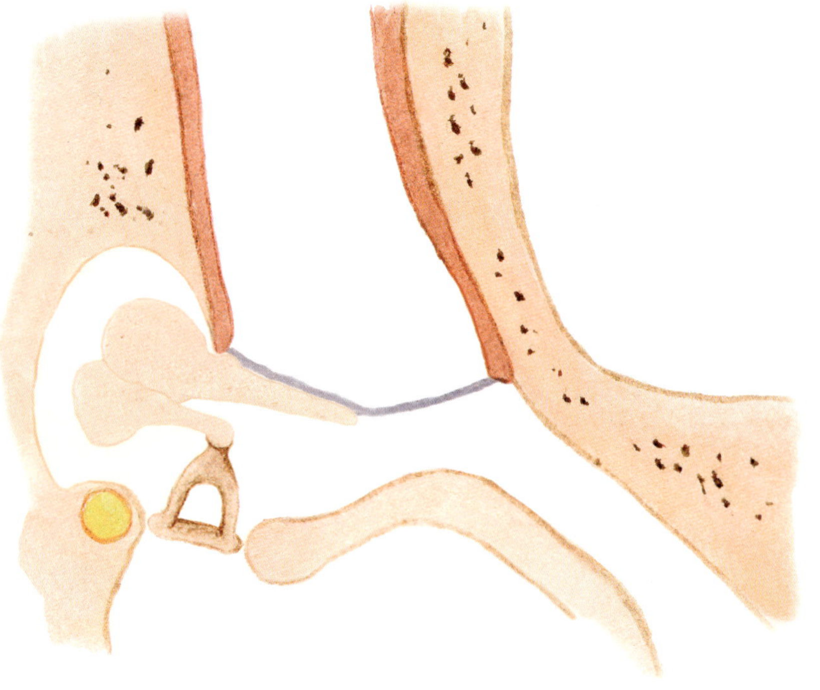

Fig. 5.1

Type 2 Tympanoplasty

Any ossiculoplasty involving the stapes with a columella effect from the stapes to the malleus handle or eardrum (intact or reconstructed).
Fig. 5.2

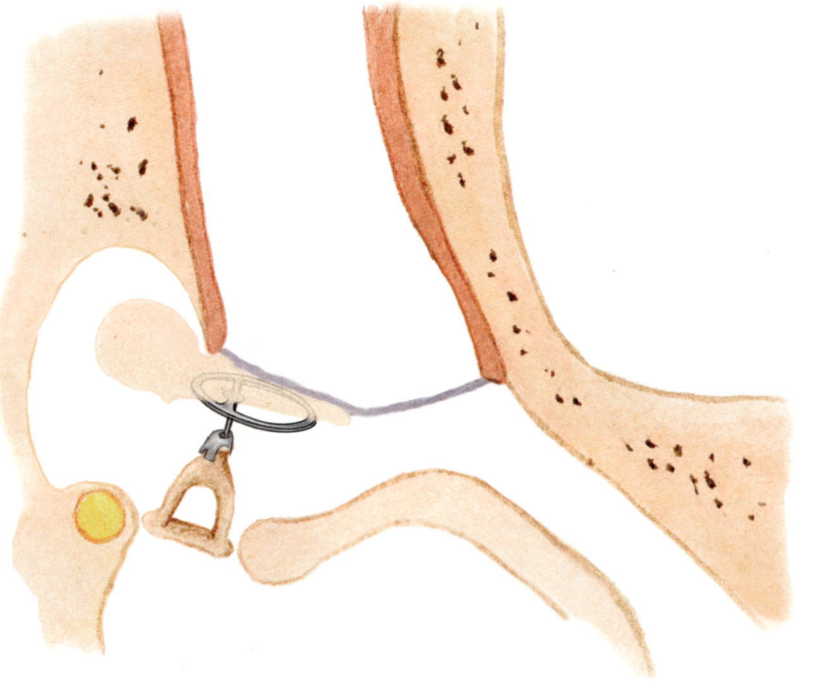

Fig. 5.2

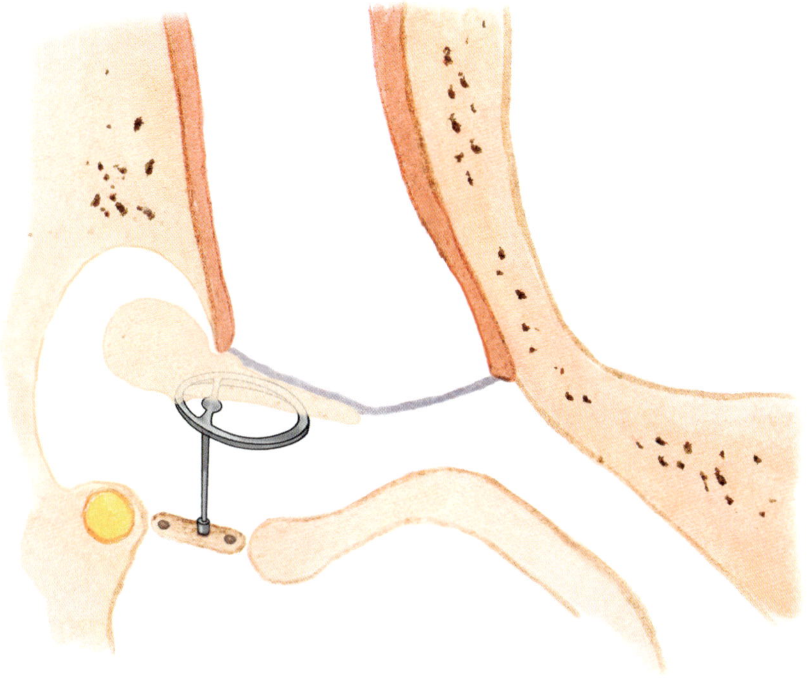

Fig. 5.3

Type 3 Tympanoplasty

Reconstruction in case of an absent or severely defective stapes. The columella extends from the footplate to the malleus handle or eardrum (intact or reconstructed).

Fig. 5.3

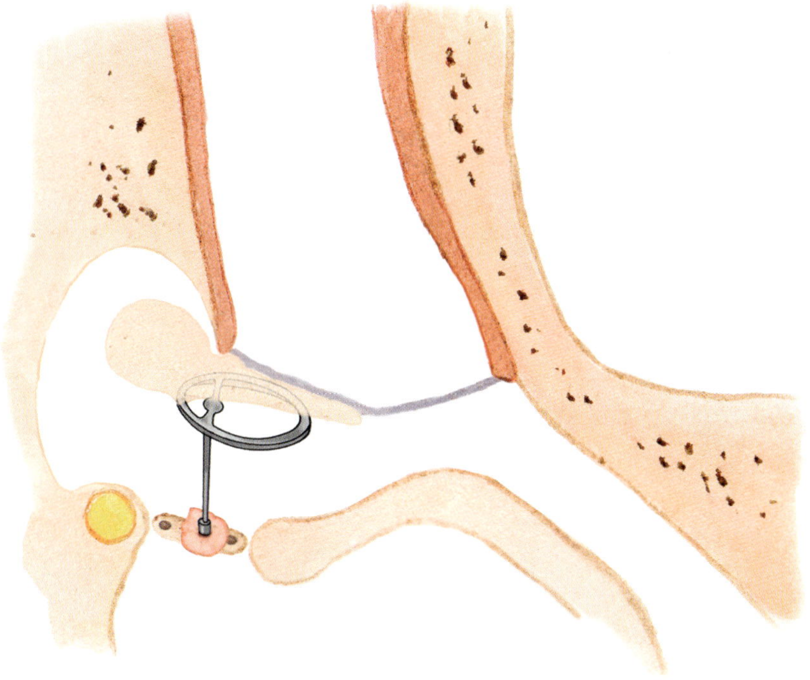

Fig. 5.4

Type 4 Tympanoplasty

Platinotomy for a fixed footplate and no ossicles (except malleus). The eardrum must be intact.

Fig. 5.4

Fixation of the Intact Chain

Malleus and Incus Fixation

The incus or malleus can be fixed in the epitympanic region.

Fig. 5.5

The fixation approach usually involves posterior epitympanotomy (see Posterior Epitympanotomy, p. 119). It requires careful drilling with a diamond burr on the approach to the short process of the incus. If the incudomallear complex is not visible enough and safe access not guaranteed, the incus is removed by the transcanal route.

Incus Removal

After dislocation of the incudostapedial joint with a small round knife or microhook, the incus is lateralized using a small hook. The long process of the incus is grasped with microforceps (see Removal of the Incus, p. 90).

Small anteroposterior movements allow the incudomallear joint to be freed, before the incus is pulled inferiorly and removed.

Fig. 5.6

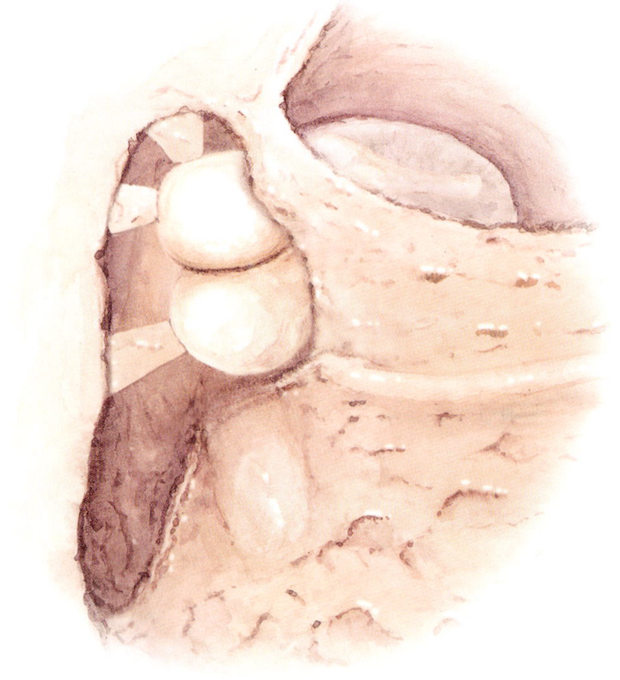

Fig. 5.5

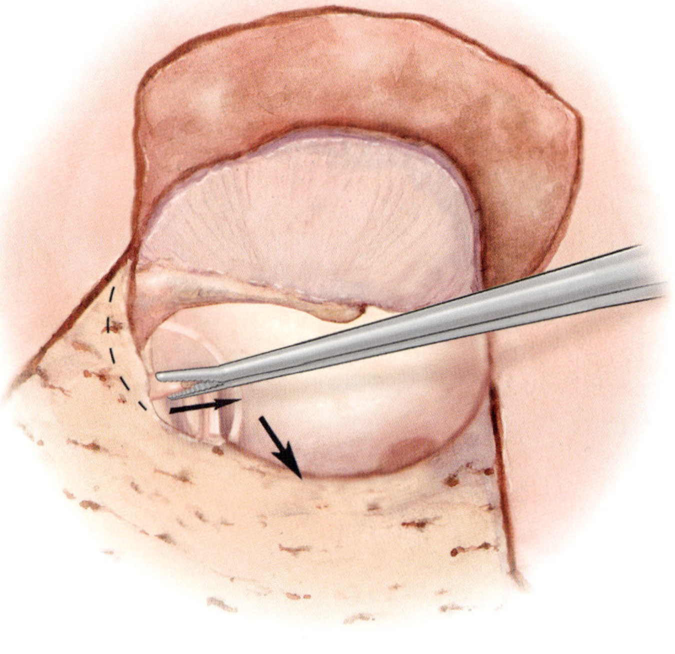

Fig. 5.6

Malleus Head Removal
If the malleus remains fixed, the malleus head must be removed using a malleus head nipper before type 2 ossiculoplasty is performed (see also pp. 92–97).

Fig. 5.7

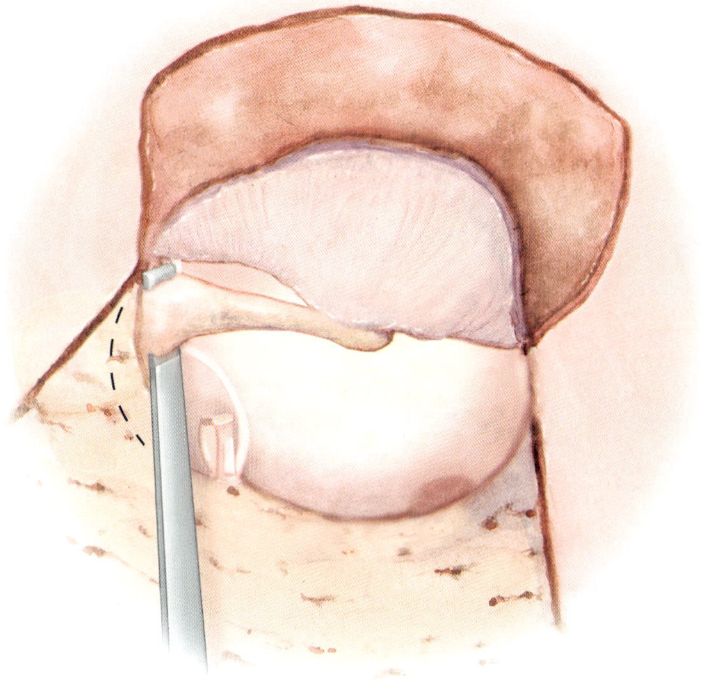

Fig. 5.7

Malleus Tendon Cut
If malleus handle movement is still compromised, the malleus tendon may be calcified and should be cut using curved or straight microscissors.

If there is sufficient exposure, the bony fixation of the incus or malleus head can be drilled using a very thin diamond burr. Adequate space should be created between the ossicle and bony wall to avoid recurrence of fixation. A Silastic sheet may be inserted in between.

Fig. 5.8

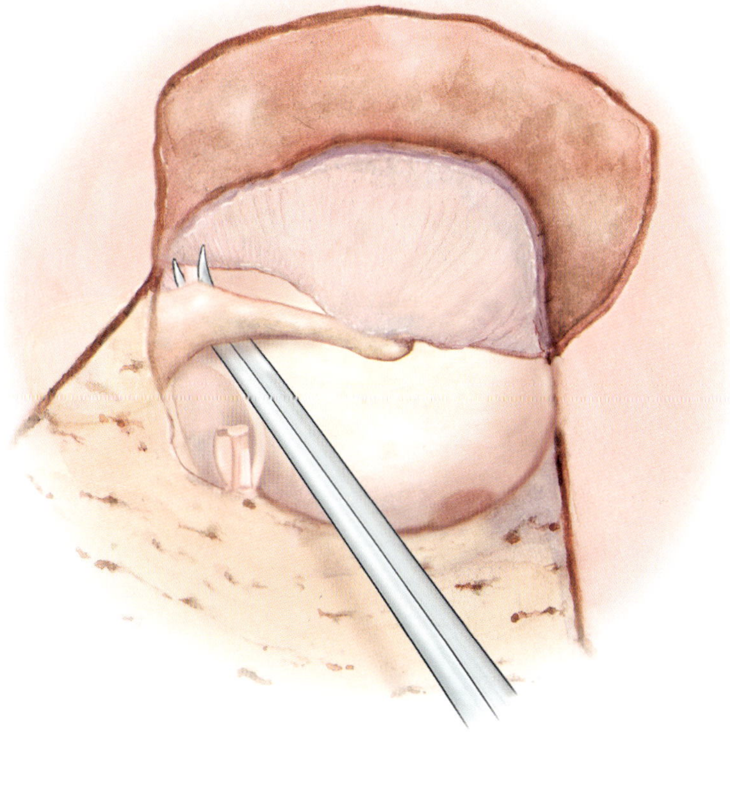

Fig. 5.8

Stapes Fixation in Tympanosclerosis

The stapes may be fixed by tympanosclerotic plaques. The tympanic membrane must be intact to manage stapes immobility. Tympanosclerotic plaques can be carefully removed using a needle or small hook. Stapes mobility can be restored, but refixation frequently occurs. Generally, the superstructure should be removed using a laser or microscissors. The footplate is cleaned of the tympanosclerosis with a needle or small hook, moving parallel to the facial nerve in an anteroposterior direction. Footplate mobility is thus restored and an ossiculoplasty is performed. If the footplate remains fixed, a stapedotomy is performed.

Tip: The hearing and pathological status of the contralateral ear and bone conduction of the operated ear has to be considered before a stapedotomy is performed. Inner ear damage is more frequent with tympanosclerosis than with otosclerosis. Classic or specific implantable hearing aids can be a safe alternative (e. g., the Vibrant Soundbridge [Med-el, Innsbruck, Austria] plugged into the round window).

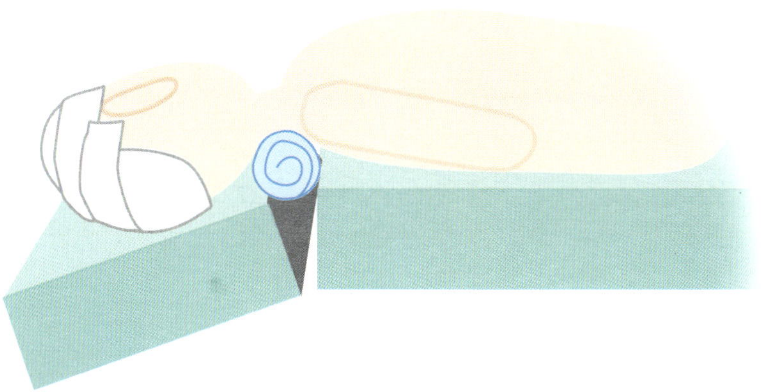

Fig. 5.9

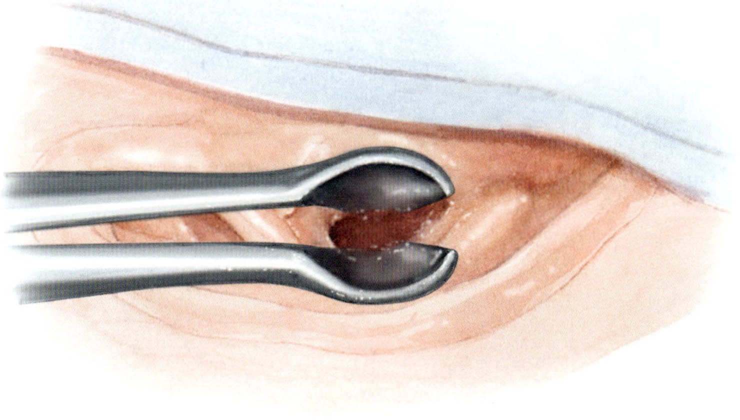

Fig. 5.10

Stapes Fixation in Otosclerosis

In our experience, a transcanal approach is used in 98 % of all surgical procedures. In the case of a very narrow external auditory canal or second-stage surgery for stapedial tympanosclerosis, however, a retroauricular approach is required.

Stapes Surgery, Head Position

The position of the patient's head and local anesthesia are very important to obtain an optimal view of the oval window and reduce bleeding (see Local Anesthesia, p. 8, and Surgical Field, p. 9).

Fig. 5.9

Transcanal Approach

A short nasal speculum is used until work is started on the ossicular chain. The disinfection liquid is aspirated completely and the canal is washed out with water.

Fig. 5.10

Tip: The advantages of the nasal speculum are that it makes it easy to change the operative field of vision and adapts to all canal diameters.

Skin Incision

The procedure starts with a Rosen incision, a curved incision from 12 o'clock to 6 o'clock.

A lateral incision is first made inferiorly at 6 o'clock, then superiorly at 12 o'clock, using a lateral knife. The superior incision must be at least 8–10 mm long and the inferior incision 6–8 mm.

A circumferential incision joins the lateral incisions in a curve.

Fig. 5.11

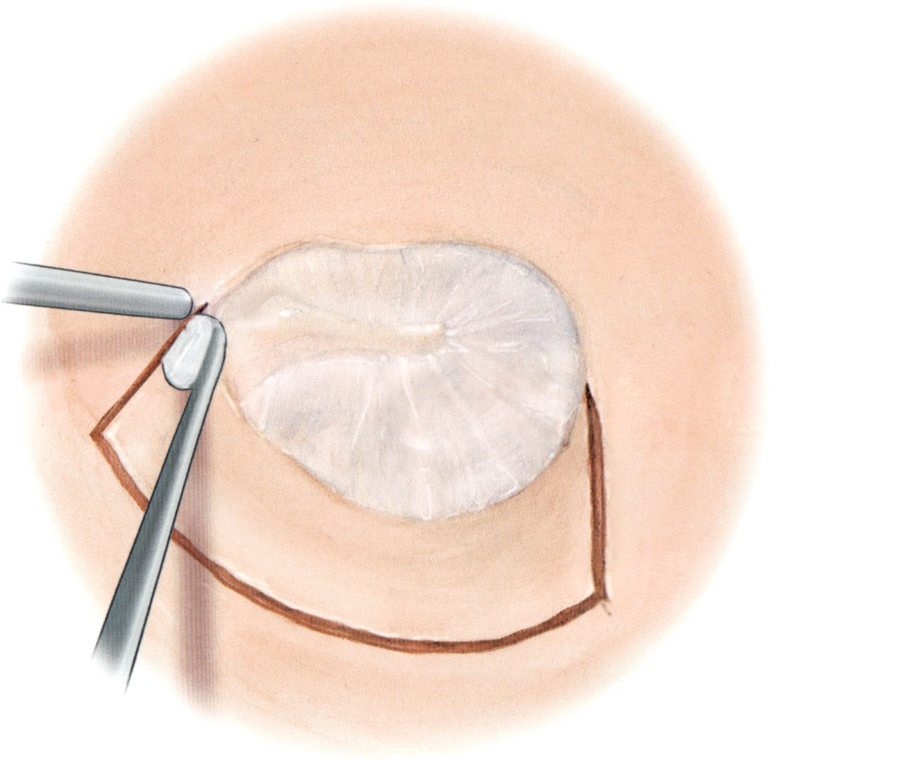

Fig. 5.11

Skin Flap Elevation

The skin flap is elevated toward the fibrous annulus using a small, round knife.

Because of the skin thickness, and to preserve smooth edges, it is sometimes necessary to complete the superolateral incision using straight microscissors.

Microsuction is performed with a small cotton ball or piece of Merocel soaked in 1 % lidocaine with 5 µg/mL epinephrine to protect the skin and reduce bleeding.

Fig. 5.12

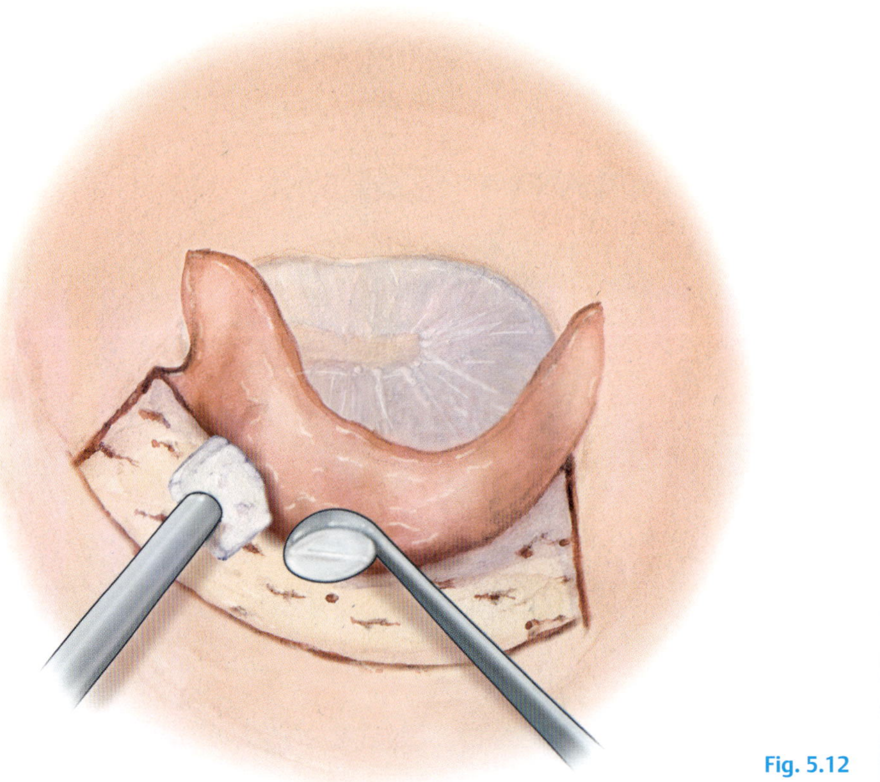

Fig. 5.12

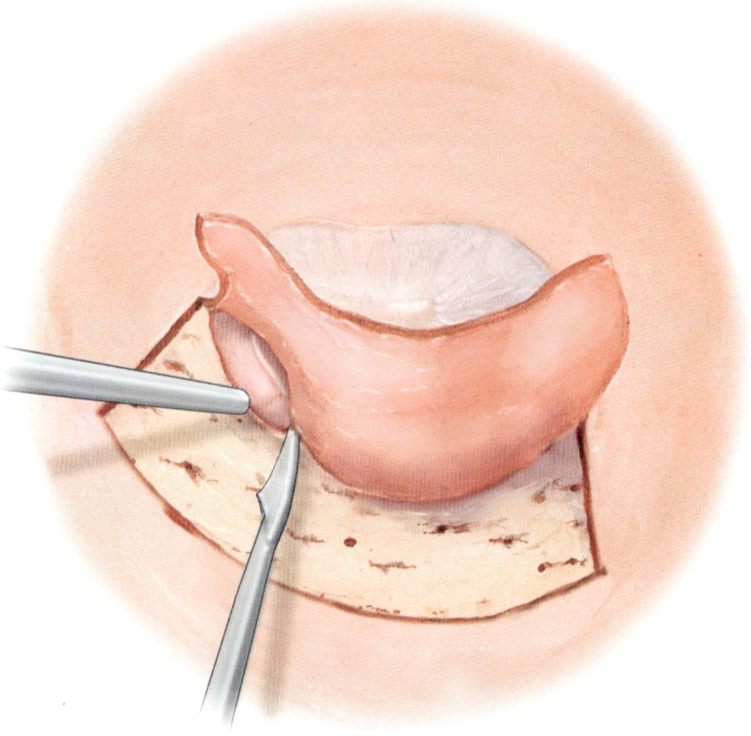

Fig. 5.13

Tympanomeatal Flap Elevation

A needle or sickle knife is inserted between the chordal eminence and short process of malleus, and the tympanic membrane is elevated. Then, using a lateral knife, the fibrous annulus is dislocated out of the sulcus starting at the transition of the chordal eminence, paying special attention to the chorda tympani. The middle ear mucosa must be incised to enter the middle ear cavity. When the opening is large enough, a flap knife or dissector-elevator is inserted and the fibrous annulus is luxated until an adequate view of the malleus neck and the round window is achieved.

Fig. 5.13

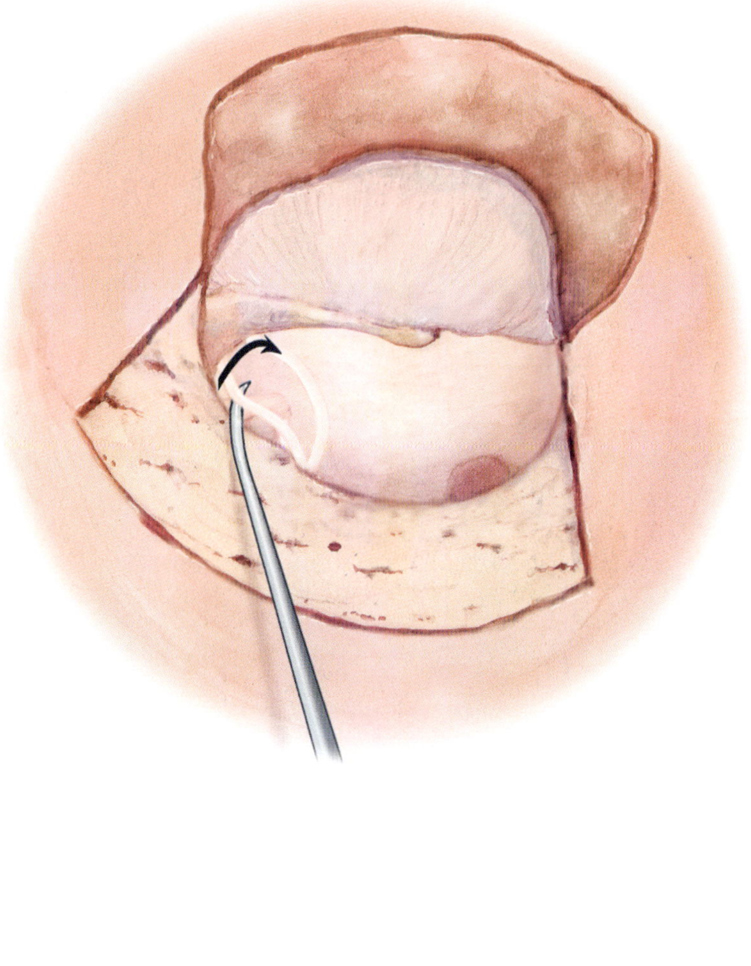

Fig. 5.14

Chorda Tympani Dissection

If the chorda tympani compromises access to the stapes and oval window, the nerve must be disinserted from its bony well using a needle or microhook.

Fig. 5.14

Chorda Tympani Mobilization

The chorda tympani is pushed medially without being stretched

Fig. 5.15

Tip: In some cases, it is necessary to perform a small posterior atticotomy prior to chorda tympani luxation with a small curette.
If it is not possible to push the chorda tympani medially, it can be pushed posteriorly. This step is sometimes performed after atticotomy.

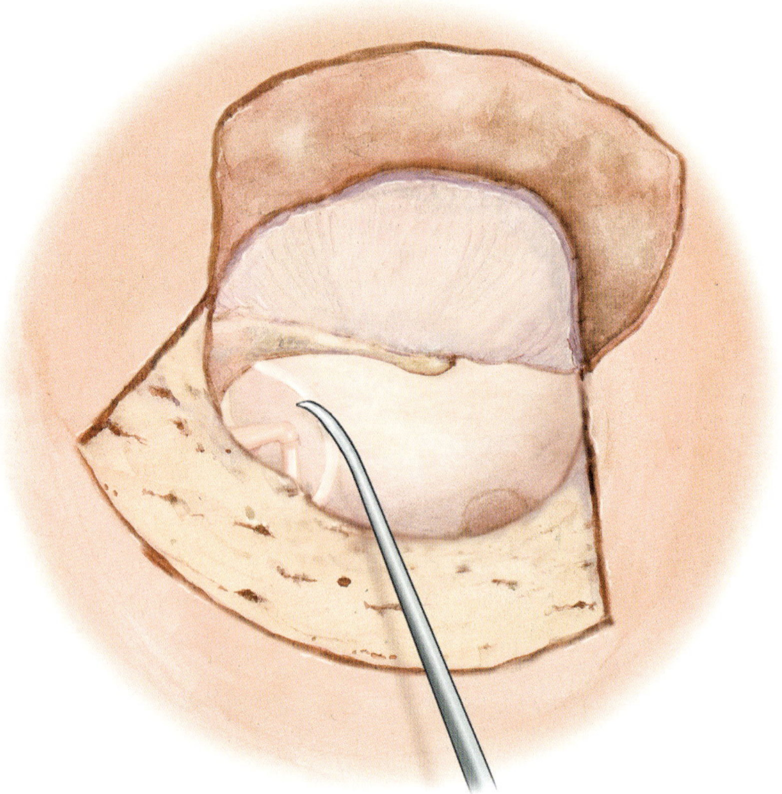

Fig. 5.15

Posterior Tympanoatticotomy

Bony Frame Fracture

Tympanoatticotomy is performed using a 3-mm chisel. The bone is fractured perpendicularly and tangentially to the frame.

Fig. 5.16

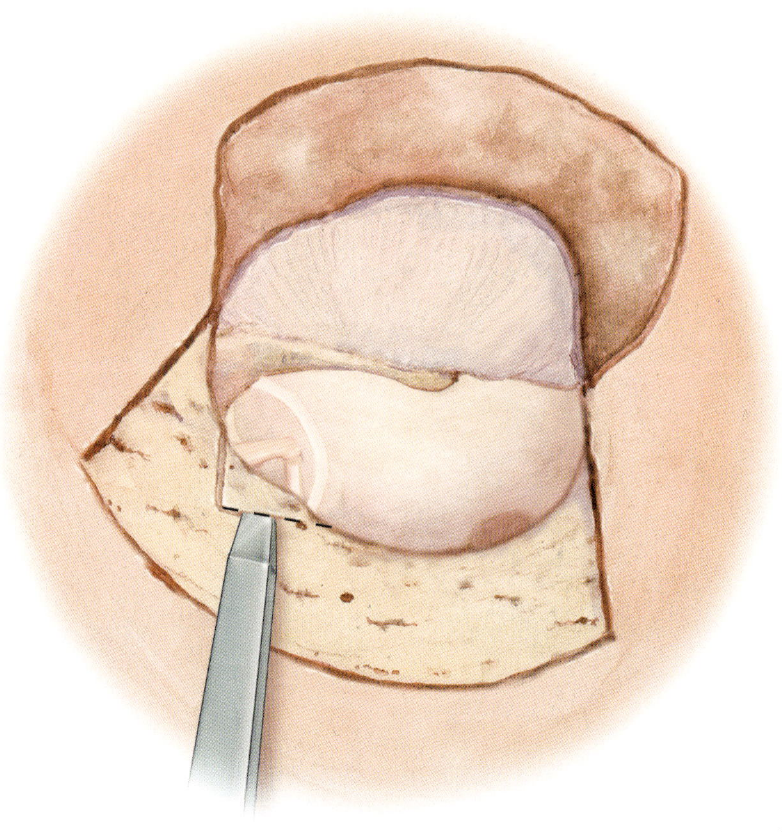

Fig. 5.16

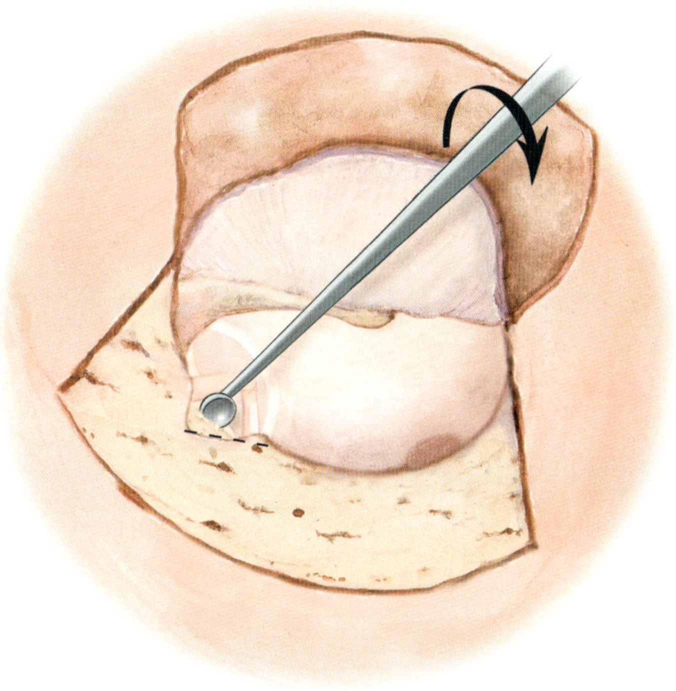

Fig. 5.17

Atticotomy Optimalization

The atticotomy is completed with a curette to expose two-thirds of the long process of the incus, the facial nerve above the oval window, the oval window itself, the posterior crus of the stapes, and the stapedial tendon and pyramidal eminence. The curette is applied using posterior and inferior rotation movements.

Fig. 5.17

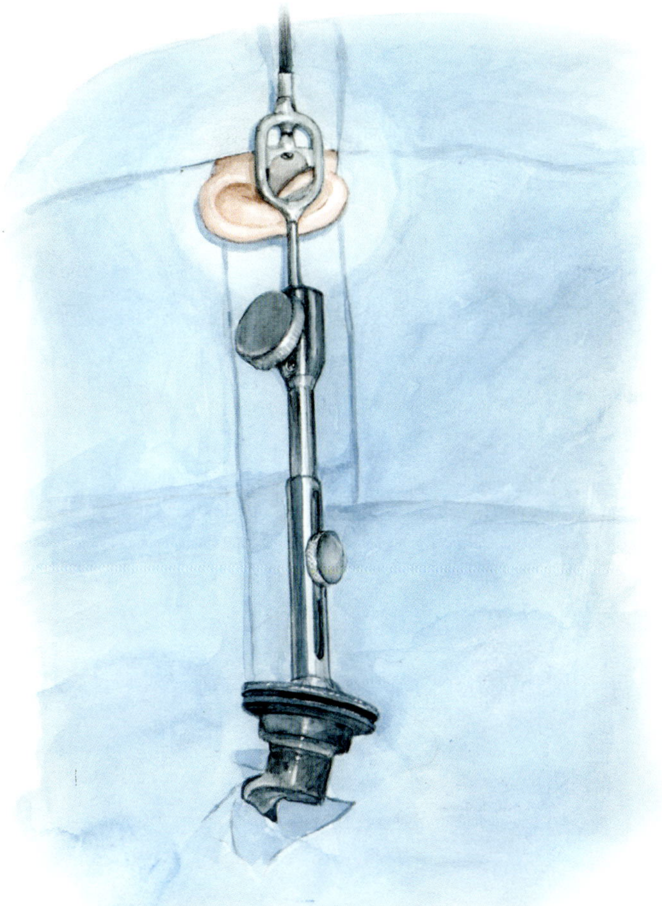

Fig. 5.18

Placement of a Portmann Retractor

Placement of a Portmann retractor allows a bimanual technique to be used. An adequate view of the structures previously described is vital. To this end, the atticotomy must be sufficiently large, rotation of the patient's head must be adjusted, and the speculum must be positioned perpendicular to the canal and opened as wide as possible.

Fig. 5.18

Checking Fixation of the Ossicular Chain and Facial Nerve

Malleus and Incus Mobility Testing

Mobility of the ossicular chain is checked using a needle. The malleus handle is gently pulled up to verify the integrity and mobility of the incudomallear complex.

Fig. 5.19

Malleus or Incus Fixation and Stapes Mobility Testing

In the case of fixation, the incus is removed with or without the malleus head. A different type of prosthesis is then used (see Major Discontinuity of the Incudostapedial Joint Stapes Useful, p. 90). The stapes fixation is checked.

Facial Nerve Position

Facial nerve position and abnormalities are identified. The nerve might be partially or totally uncovered, protruding, or it may present anatomical variations. Adapted maneuvers or careful use of laser should be considered in such circumstances.

Disarticulation of the Incudostapedial Joint

Using a small, round knife or small hook, the incudostapedial joint is totally disarticulated. Pulling up the long process of the incus helps to locate the joint. The instrument slowly slices through the articulation using small rotational movements.

Fig. 5.20

Tip: If the joint cannot be identified, pull the long process of the incus laterally with a small hook to reveal the exact position of the joint.

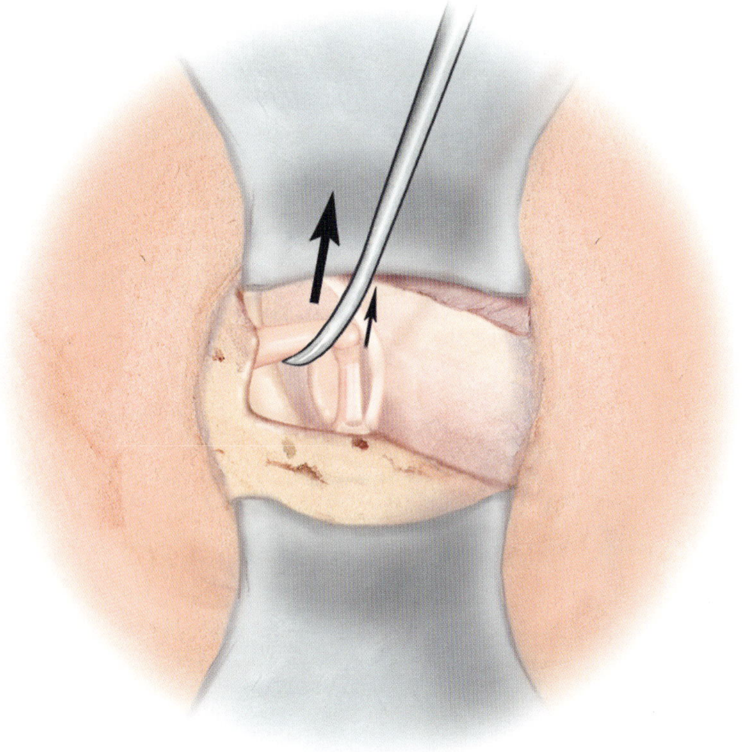

Fig. 5.19

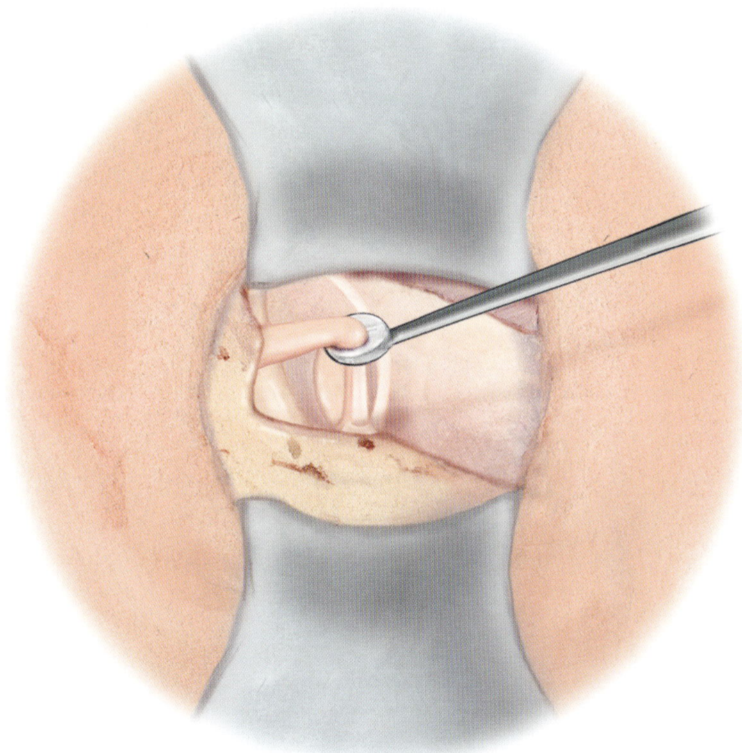

Fig. 5.20

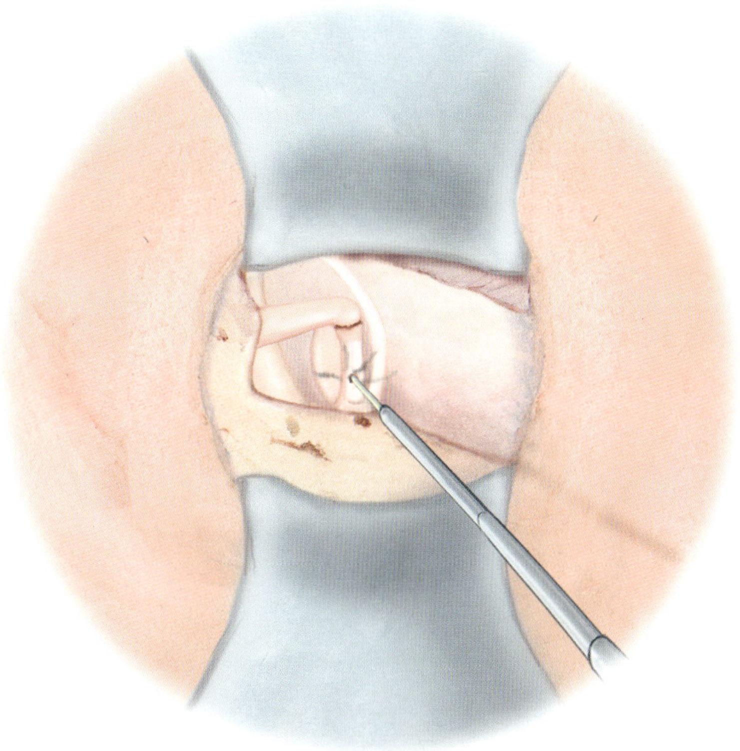

Fig. 5.21

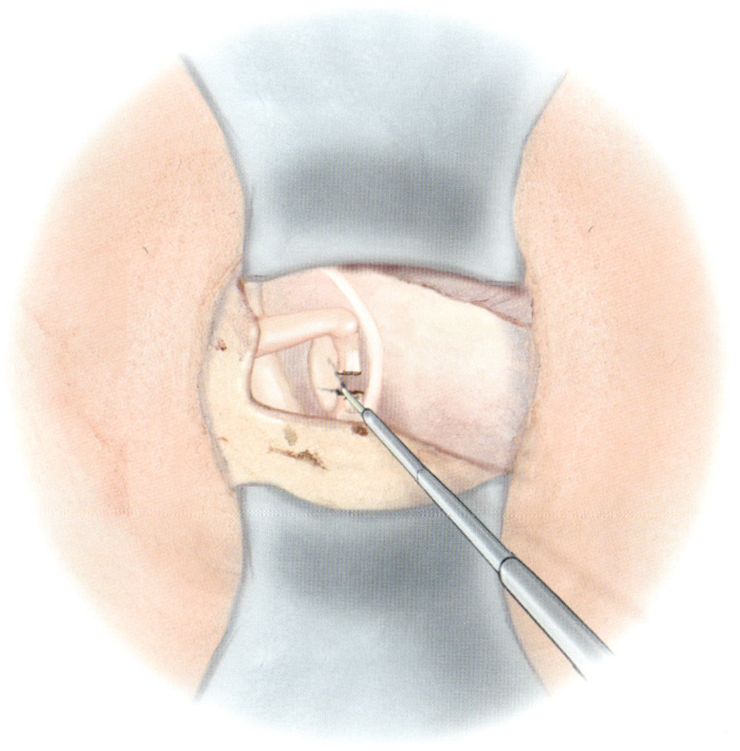

Fig. 5.22

Removal of the Stapes Superstructure

Stapedial Tendon Cut

The stapedial tendon is cut with straight microscissors or a diode laser (1.5 W in continuous mode). Section of the tendon exposes the posterior crus.

Fig. 5.21

Posterior Crus Cut

A diode laser is applied to cut the posterior crus in its inferior half. The protruding pyramidal eminence can be drilled using a Skeeter drill (Medtronic Xomed). A diamond or cutting microburr of 0.6–1 mm is utilized. Use of a diamond microburr minimizes bleeding.

Fig. 5.22

Tip: A diode laser (808–940 nm) is a visible-spectrum laser. Its characteristics are similar to those of the KTP laser with high water diffusion inducing a higher theoretical risk of inner ear and facial nerve damage. Other types of laser other than the diode laser can be used. It is important to know the properties of each individual laser, as this helps to avoid complications. A diode laser has high water diffusion. It should be use on a dry surface to reduce heat diffusion.

Anterior Crus Cut

The anterior crus is generally hidden by the long process of the incus. Rotation of the patient's head might facilitate visualization and allow its section using the diode laser. In the majority of cases, the anterior crus is identified by touching it with the laser probe. It is broken blindly.
Fig. 5.23

Stapes Superstructure Removal

Sometimes this step is not possible and the anterior crus is broken up by means of small left-to-right lateral movements of the superstructure with a needle or microhook. When the superstructure feels free, it is pushed onto the promontory to be removed using fine microforceps.
Fig. 5.24

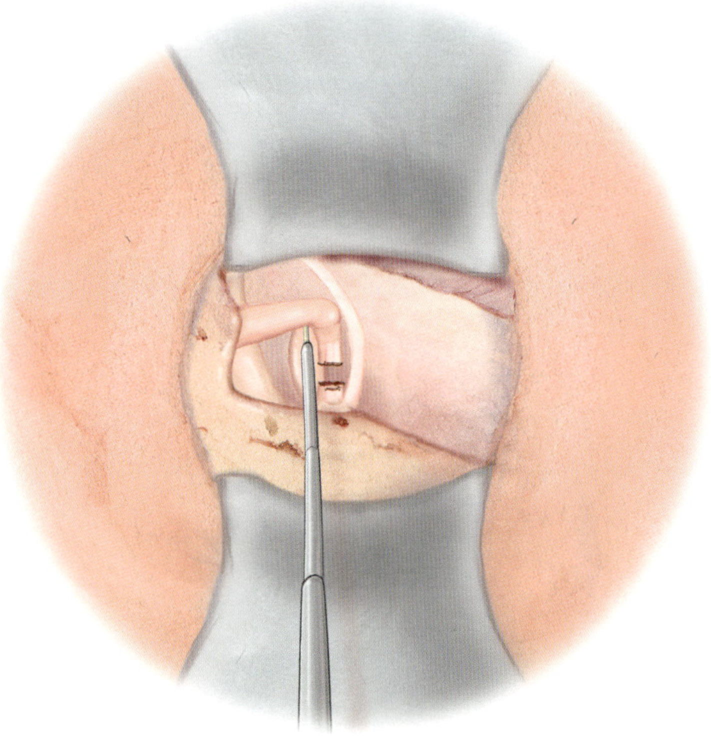

Fig. 5.23

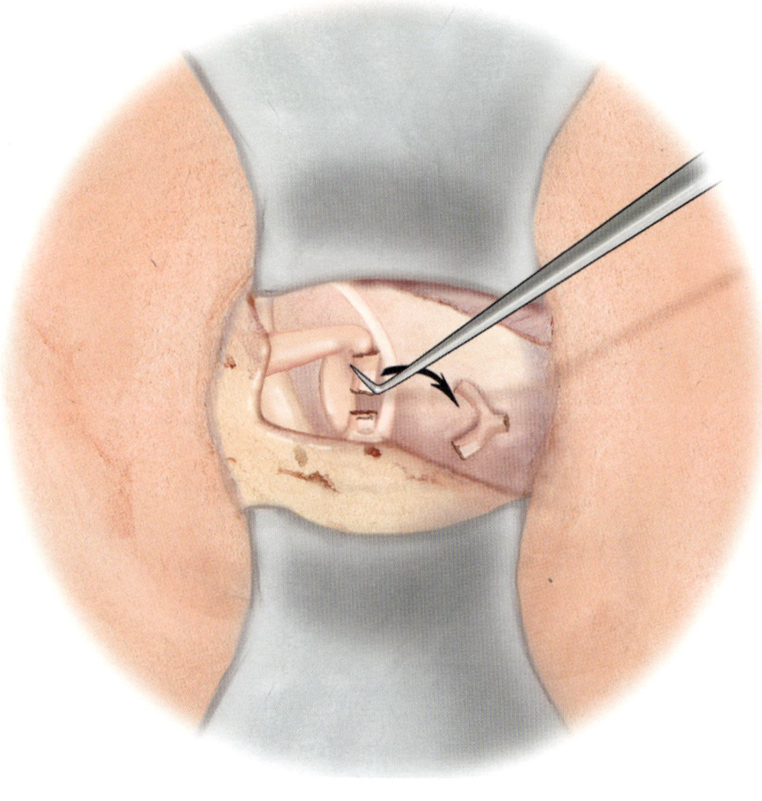

Fig. 5.24

Grade of Otosclerosis (according to Portmann and Guerrier 1986)

Grade I

Normal appearance of the footplate, but with ligament ankylosis

Fig. 5.25

Grade II:

Small ankylosed region of the anterior part of the footplate

Fig. 5.26

Grade III

Large ankylosed region (>50%) of the footplate surface

Fig. 5.27

Grade IV

Totally ankylosed footplate with identified footplate limits

Fig. 5.28

Grade V:

Is the same as grade IV but without identified footplate limits.

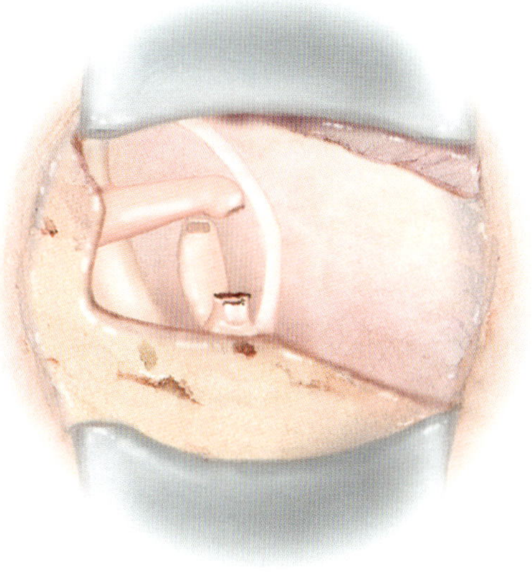

Fig. 5.25

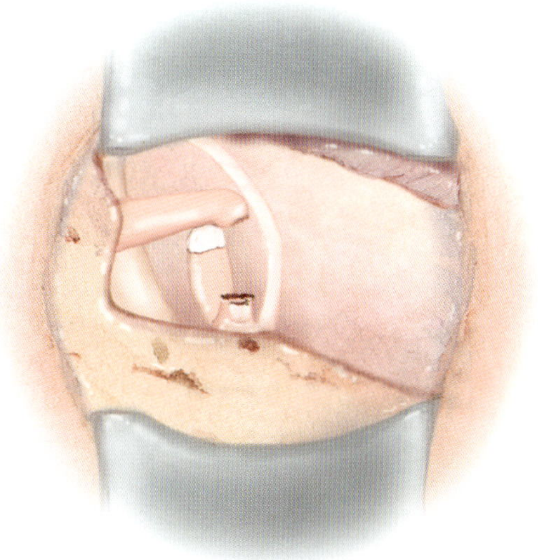

Fig. 5.26

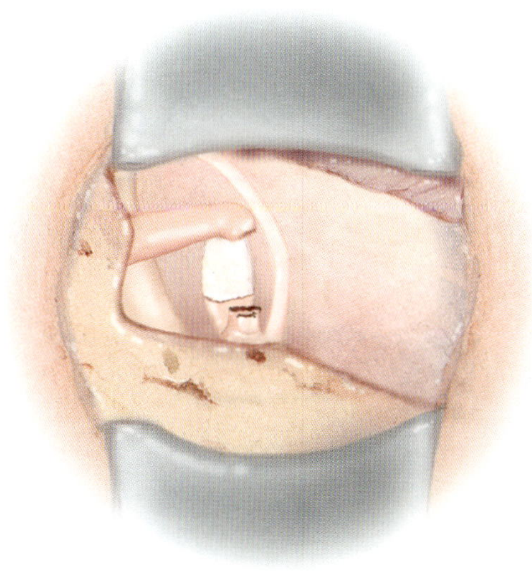

Fig. 5.27

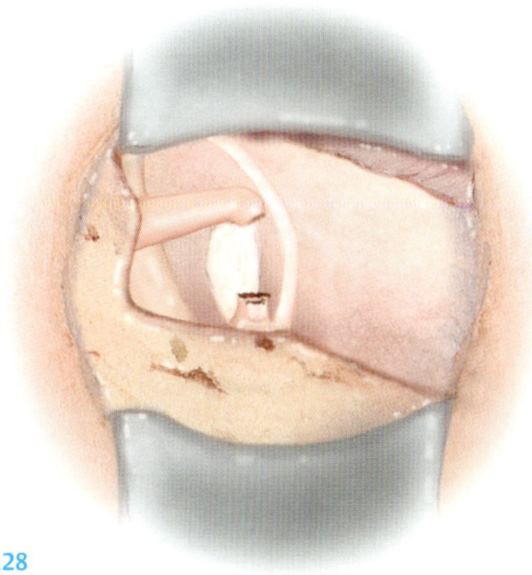

Fig. 5.28

Measurement of the Piston

A measuring rod allows evaluation of the distance between the footplates and the lateral surface of the incus. Ninety-two percent of our pistons are between 4.25 and 4.75 mm in size.

Fig. 5.29

Tip: If piston length cannot be accurately evaluated, a 4.5-mm piston will fit and be safe in most cases.

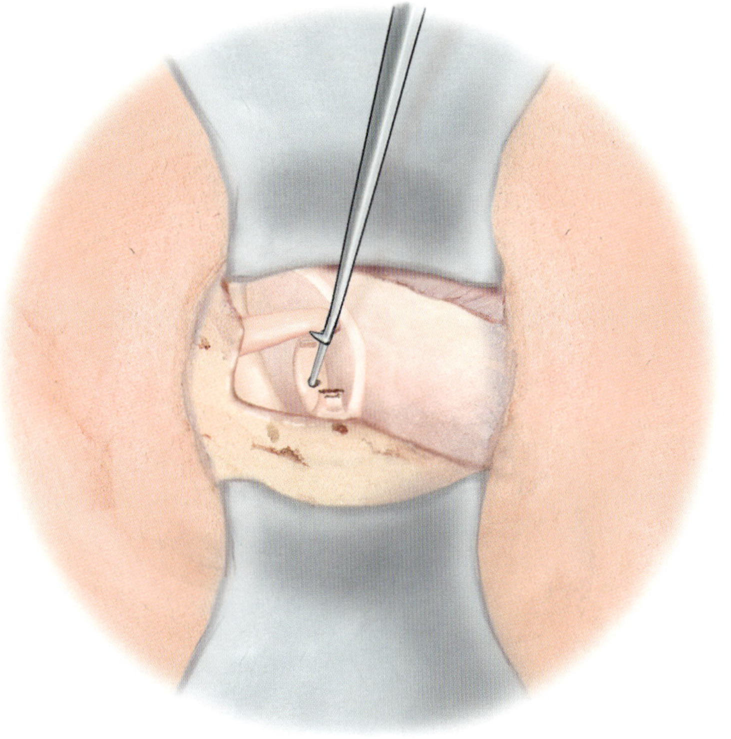

Fig. 5.29

Calibrated Stapedotomy

This technique was previously described by J. B. Causse and colleagues (Vincent et al. 1996).

Because of the technique used (laser shattering and microdrill stapedotomy), the calibrated stapedotomy can be performed after superstructure removal.

Footplate Shattering

Using the diode laser probe (1 W in continuous mode), the footplate is shattered in its posterior third, or in the center in difficult, unreachable cases. This helps to prevent bleeding.

Fig. 5.30

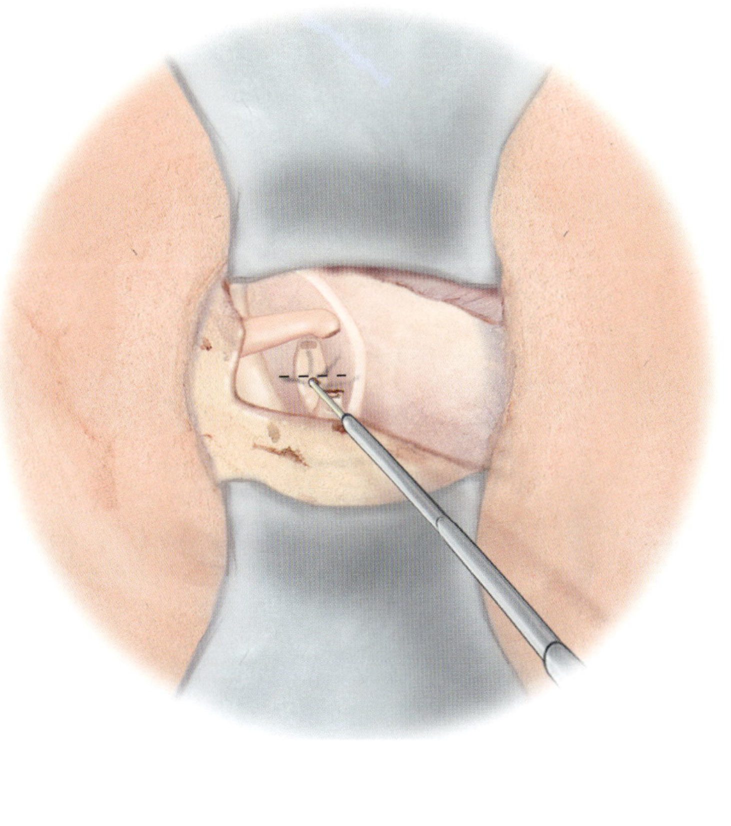

Fig. 5.30

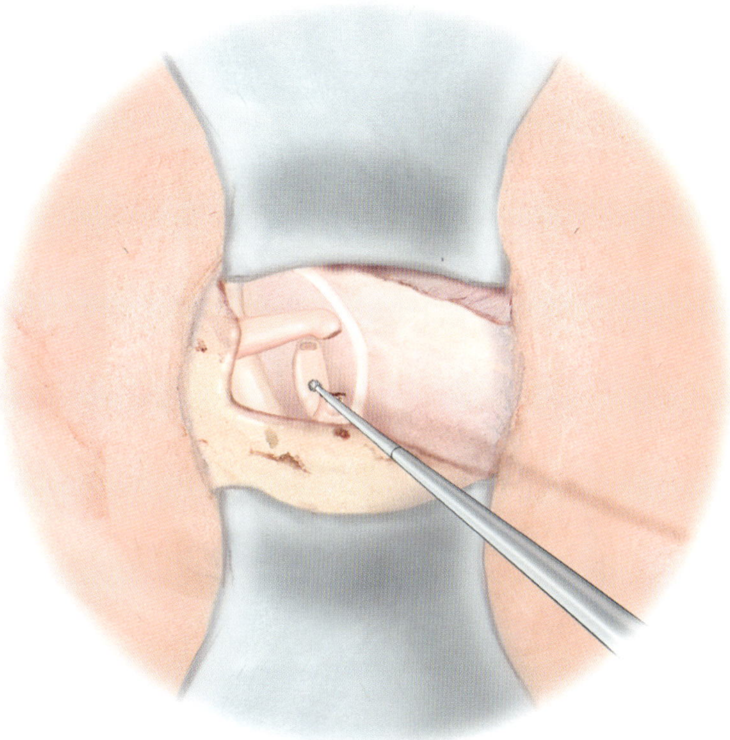

Fig. 5.31

Footplate Opening

A 0.5-mm-diameter cutting burr (0.1 mm larger than the piston) is positioned on the burned area of the footplate, and the footplate is drilled until a loss of resistance is perceived. At this moment, the drill is withdrawn and drilling stopped.

Fig. 5.31

Stapedotomy Calibration

The stapedotomy diameter can be checked with a disconnected 0.4-mm suction. Suction can never be applied directly to the stapedotomy.

Fig. 5.32

Tip: The characteristics of the diode laser give rise to a higher theoretical risk of inner ear damage. This is why the fiberoptic probe is only used to shatter the footplate, helping to reduce bleeding. The microdrill allows a perfectly calibrated platinotomy Only a 0.4-mm or 0.7-mm diameter suction should be used on the footplate. Do not aspirate on or in the footplate hole.

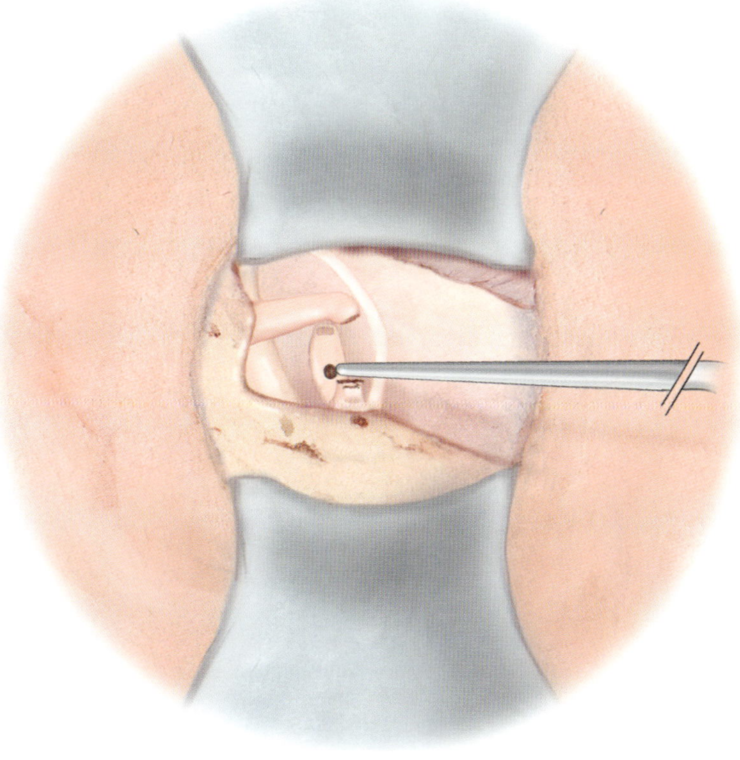

Fig. 5.32

Preparation of the Piston

A Teflon piston (Gyrus, Southborough, Massachusetts, USA) is used in the majority of cases, but other types of titanium prostheses (e.g., Big Easy Piston, Medtronic ENT, Jacksonville, Florida, USA) may be considered.

Piston Trimming

The Teflon piston is trimmed to the appropriate size on a designated cutting board.

Fig. 5.33

Loop Opening

The loop is opened with thin microforceps in both directions to avoid asymmetric memory and premature closure.

Fig. 5.34

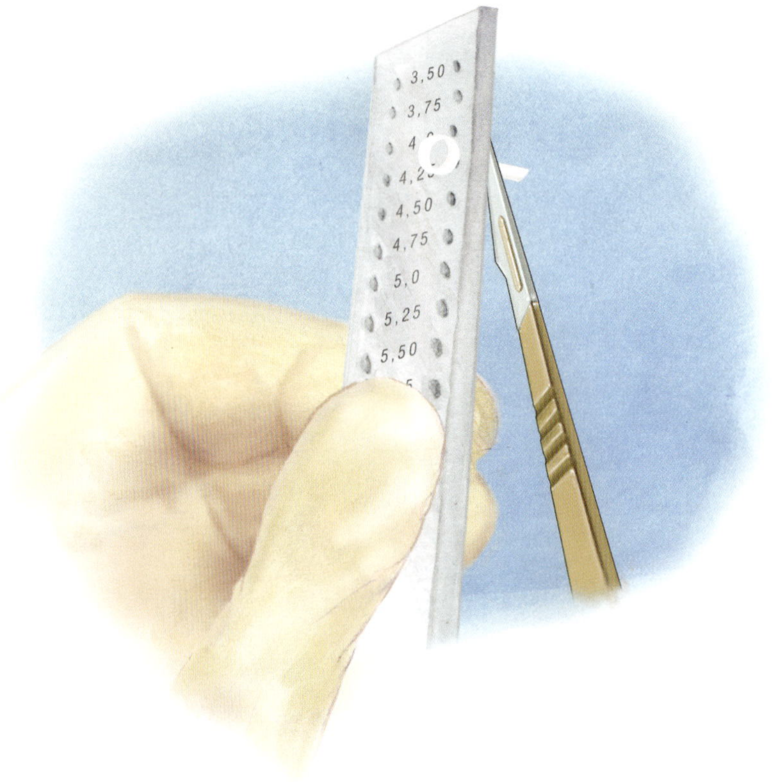

Fig. 5.33

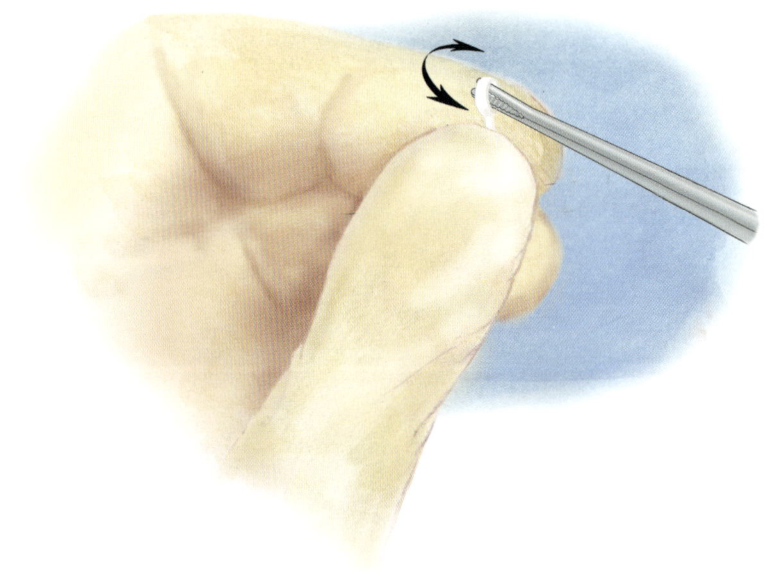

Fig. 5.34

Piston Adjustment
The piston is then placed on the thin microforceps on the posterior side of the loop facing in the same direction as the forceps or with a slightly posterior inclination.
Fig. 5.35

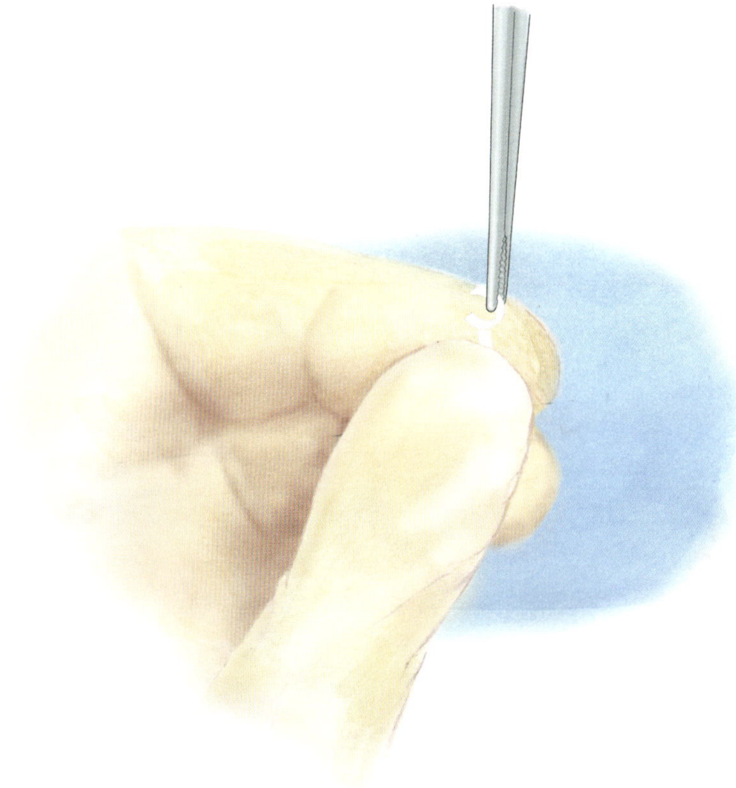

Fig. 5.35

Placement of the Piston

Reducing the focus of the microscope provides a better three-dimensional view of the platinotomy and the long process of the incus.

The piston is placed (1) in the platinotomy and (2) simultaneously clipped onto the long process of the incus. In difficult cases, the piston can first be positioned parallel to the long process of the incus, with its opened side facing down, and then clipped with a microhook.
Fig. 5.36

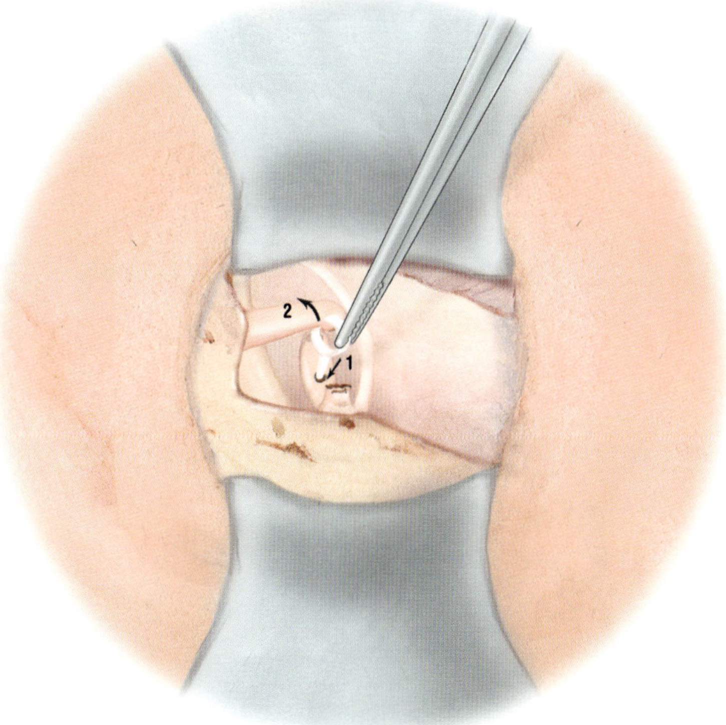

Fig. 5.36

Crimping the Piston

The piston is crimped using microforceps to allow sufficient contact without risking delayed incus erosion or fracture. The position can be adjusted with a needle and, using smooth movements, the mobility and placement of the prosthesis in the platinotomy can be evaluated.

Small pieces of Spongostan soaked in blood are placed around the piston on the footplate to stop perilymphatic leakage and guarantee prosthesis stability.

Fig. 5.37

Tympanomeatal Flap Repositioning and Packing

The tympanomeatal flap is stretched using suction and repositioned with a spatula. A simple packing with Spongostan in the canal completes the procedure.

Problems in Stapes Surgery

Obliterative Otosclerosis

In the case of a very thick footplate, laser and diamond burrs reduce more serious bleeding from the otosclerotic focus. Careful step-by-step microdrilling is essential. When the posterior half of the footplate is difficult to identify, the platinotomy should preferably be performed in the inferoposterior quadrant of the oval window.

Fig. 5.38

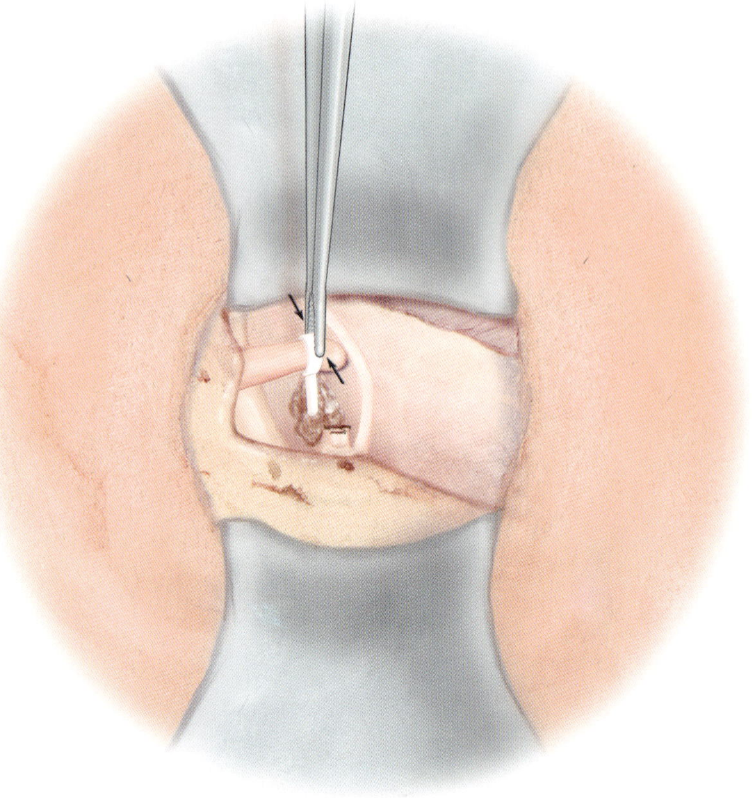

Fig. 5.37

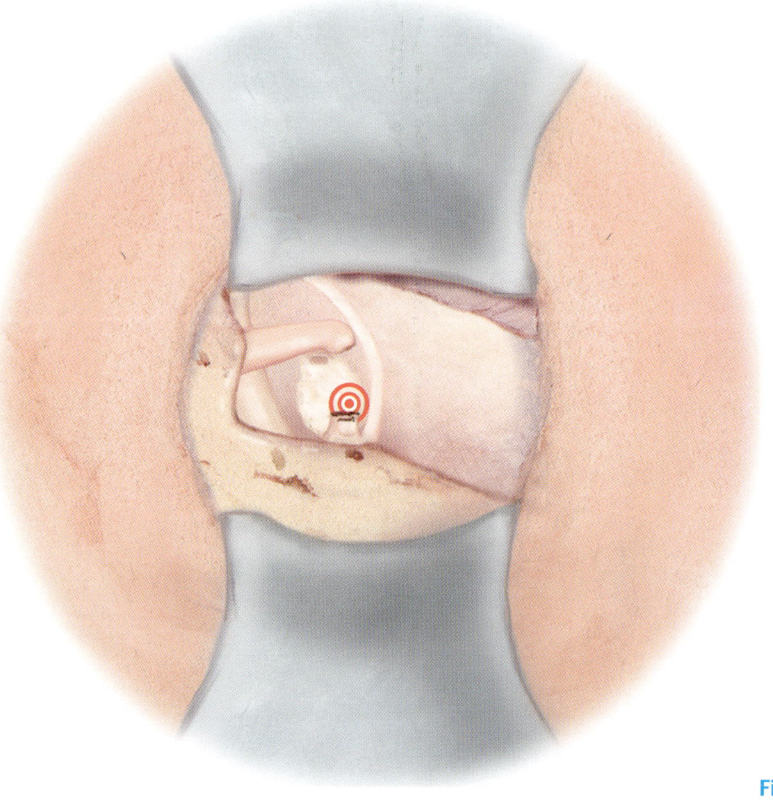

Fig. 5.38

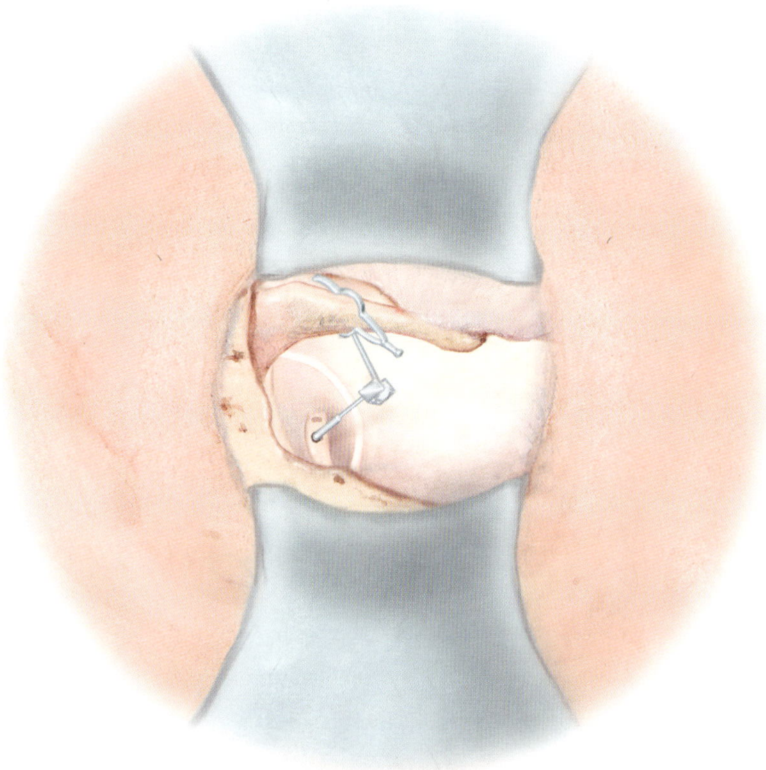

Fig. 5.39

Fixation or Significant Erosion of the Incus and Disarticulation of the Incudomallear Joint

After incus removal, mobility of the manubrium is checked. The tympanic membrane is elevated from the malleus handle (see Elevation of the Tympanic Membrane from the Malleus Handle, p. 39). A titanium MVP prosthesis (Heinz Kurz GmbH, Dusslingen, Germany) is put in place. A 6.5-mm prosthesis is generally used and its size is adjusted by modifying its articulation angle.

In the case of malleus head fixation, the fixation is removed and the same prosthesis is used.

Fig. 5.39

Difficult Approaches

In the case of a narrow external auditory canal or exostoses, a retroauricular approach is chosen. If an extensive tympanic membrane reconstruction is required, stapes surgery should be postponed until the second stage.

Shortened Long Process of the Incus or Protruding Facial Nerve

Piston Type

Use of a titanium piston (K-piston from Kurz or Big Easy from Metronic) must be considered. The prosthesis is bent to avoid contact with the facial nerve and to reach the shortened long process of the incus.

Fig. 5.40

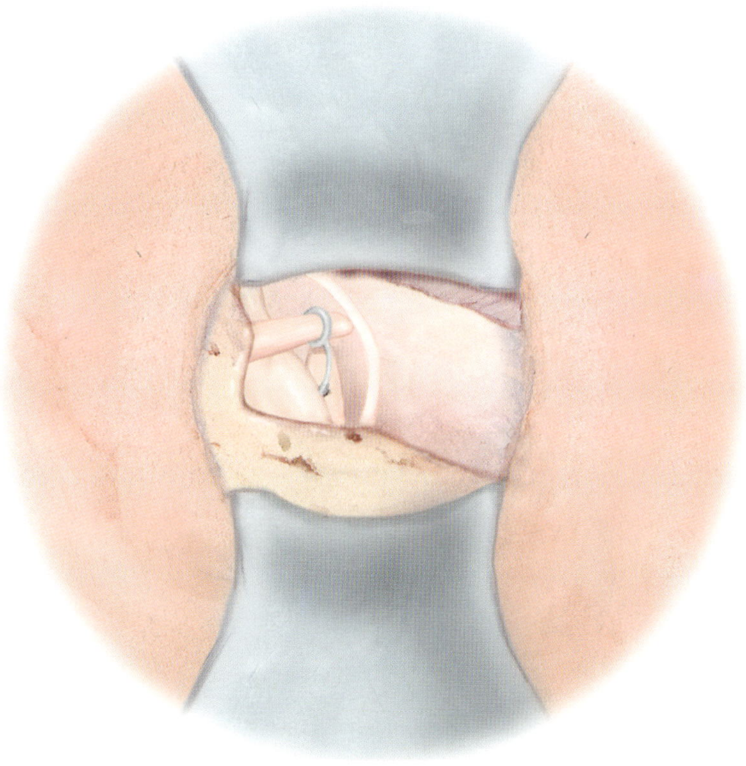

Fig. 5.40

Piston Attachment

Firm crimping of the prosthesis to the long process of the incus helps its stability. The piston fixation can be covered with a small piece of conjunctive tissue, temporalis fascia or hydroxyapatite cement.

Fig. 5.41

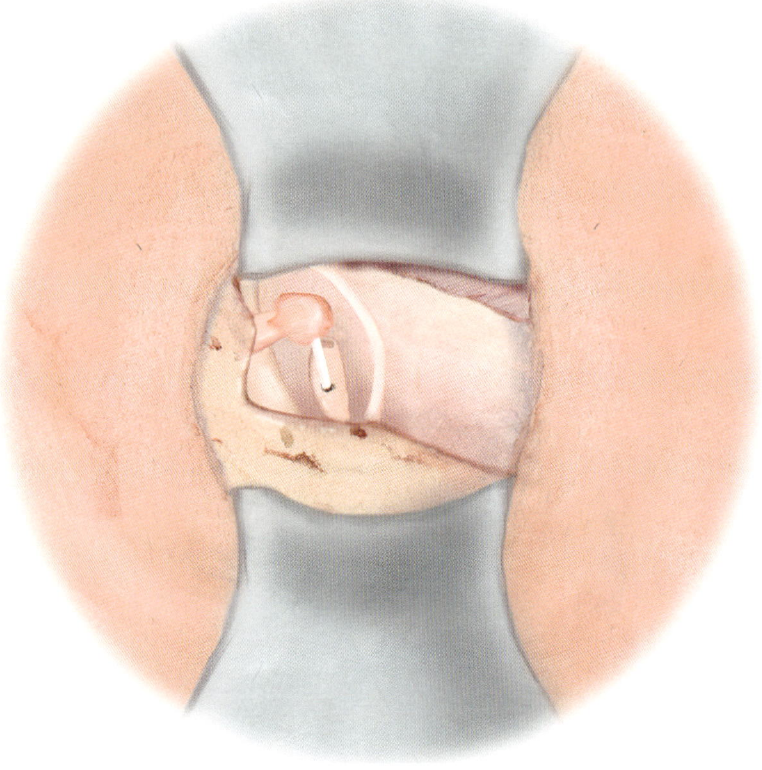

Fig. 5.41

Narrow Oval Window

When a protrusion of the facial nerve and/or promontory impedes access to the footplate, the promontory protrusion and footplate are drilled in the presumed posteroinferior area of the footplate.

Fig. 5.42

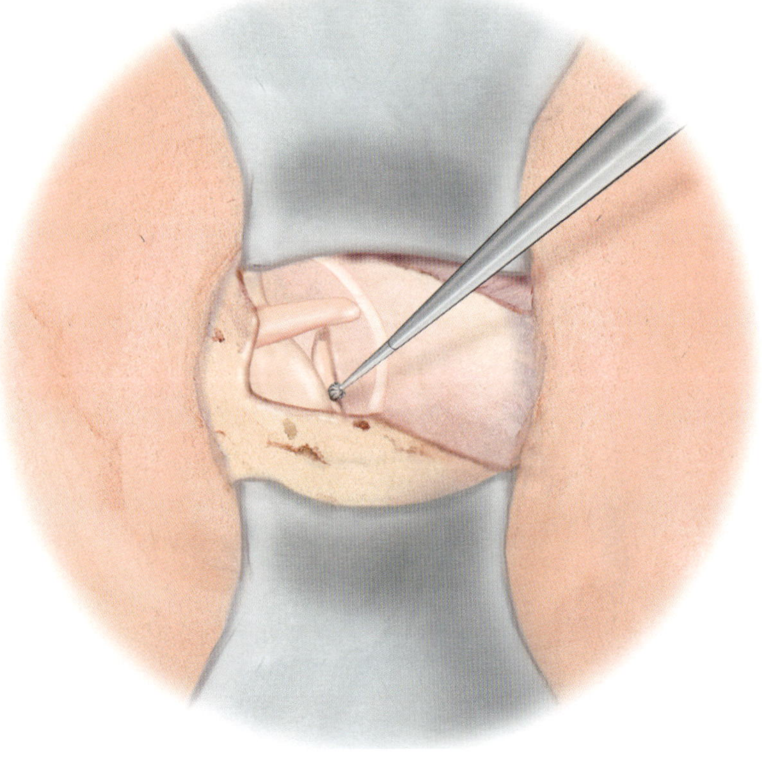

Fig. 5.42

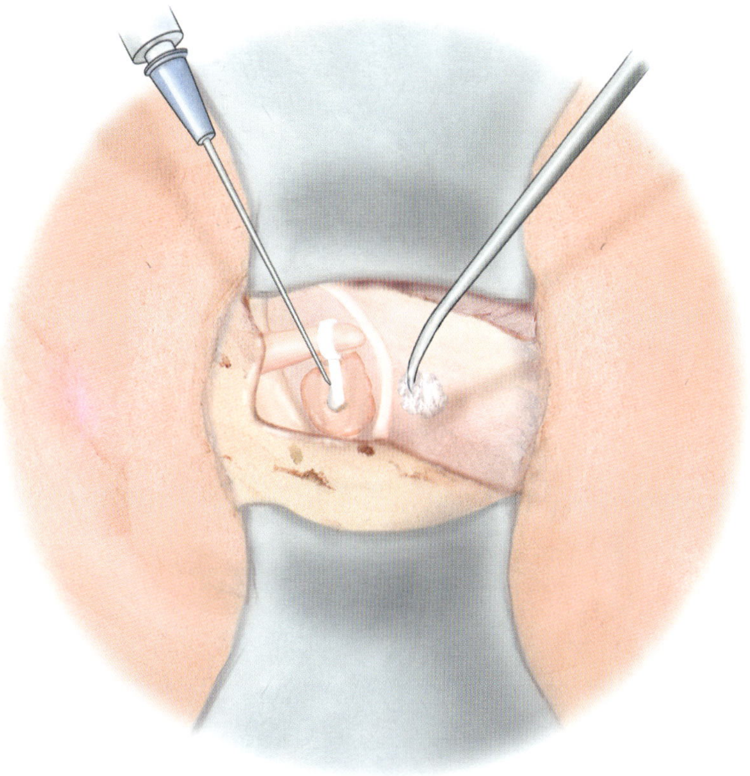

Fig. 5.43

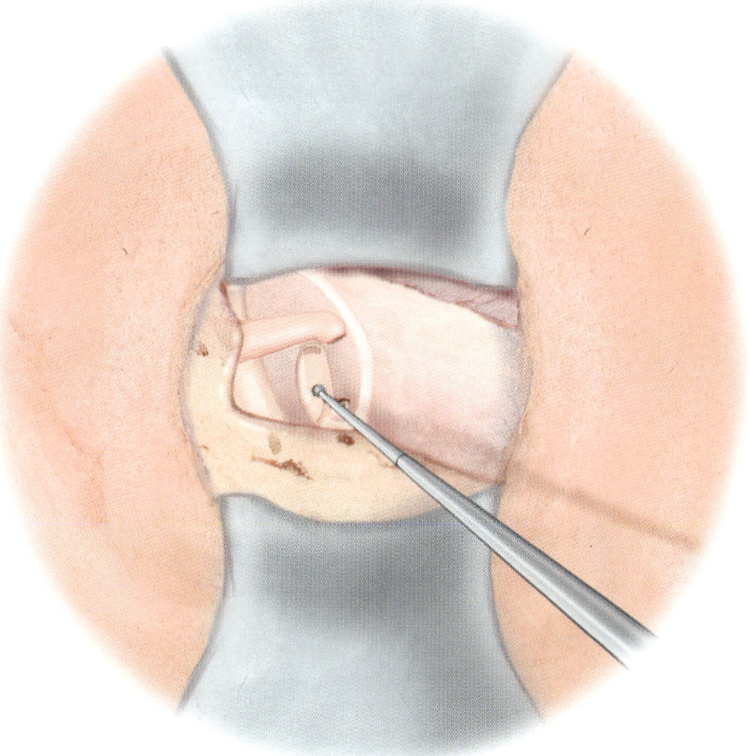

Fig. 5.44

Cerebrospinal Fluid Gusher

If cerebrospinal fluid flow is encountered, perichondrium from the posterior side of the tragus is placed over the footplate. Fibrin glue is applied and a prosthesis is positioned on the graft. A bed of Spongostan or fat from the ear lobe is packed around the prosthesis shaft.

Fig. 5.43

Tip: Even if there is a high risk of sensorineural hearing loss in such cases, placing a prosthesis helps to optimize and stabilize packing.

Floating Footplate or Stapes

The laser helps to cut the stapes branches without undue mobilization of the footplate. Both branches must be treated. A platinotomy is performed using only the laser probe (1 W in discontinuous mode). The Skeeter drill is not used. If the footplate is disrupted, it is totally or partially removed using a microhook. Tragal perichondrium interposition should be performed.

Fig. 5.44

Revision Surgery and Oval Window Management

Healing soft tissue filling the oval window should be carefully removed. When the prosthesis is removed, the newly formed membrane covering the stapedotomy is meticulously perforated with a needle and slowly opened until a sufficient diameter is obtained. In some cases, the stapedotomy needs to be enlarged using a microhook, while in extreme cases, a new stapedotomy has to be performed with a microdrill. When revision surgery is performed for a perilymphatic fistula, the oval window is filled and plugged with fat and connective tissue, and fibrin glue is added.

Disarticulation of the Intact Chain

In cases of incudomallear disarticulation, the incus is removed (see Removal of the Incus, p. 90) and type 2 ossiculoplasty is performed.

Temporalis Fascia Wrapping

Incudostapedial joint disruption can be covered with a temporalis fascia graft wrapped around the long process of the incus and stapes head.

Cement Consolidation

Biocompatible cement (hydroxyapatite cement) can be used to restore incudostapedial joint integrity. A ball of cement needs to be rubbed around the joint without any bony wall contact.

Fig. 5.45

Tip: Do not forget to check the continuity of the incudomallear complex, confirming the mobility of the reconstructed ossicular chain.

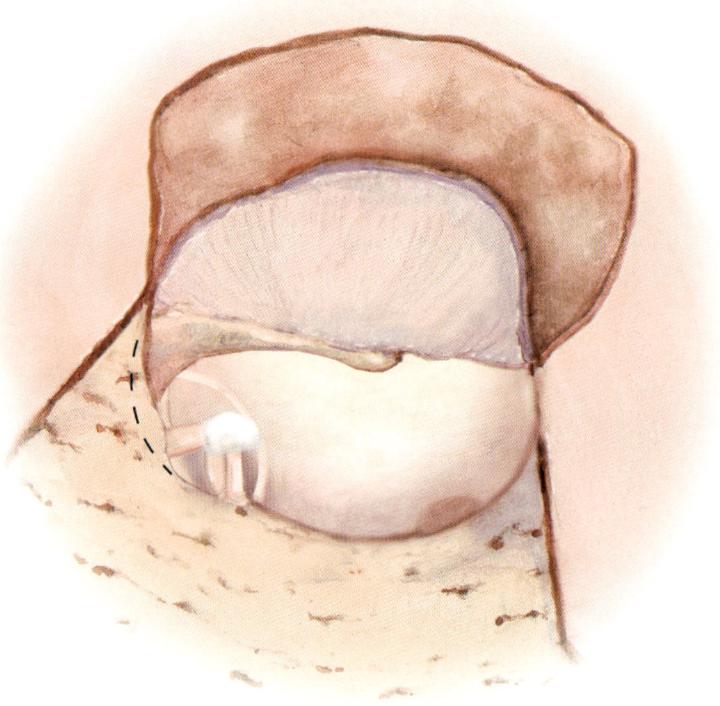

Fig. 5.45

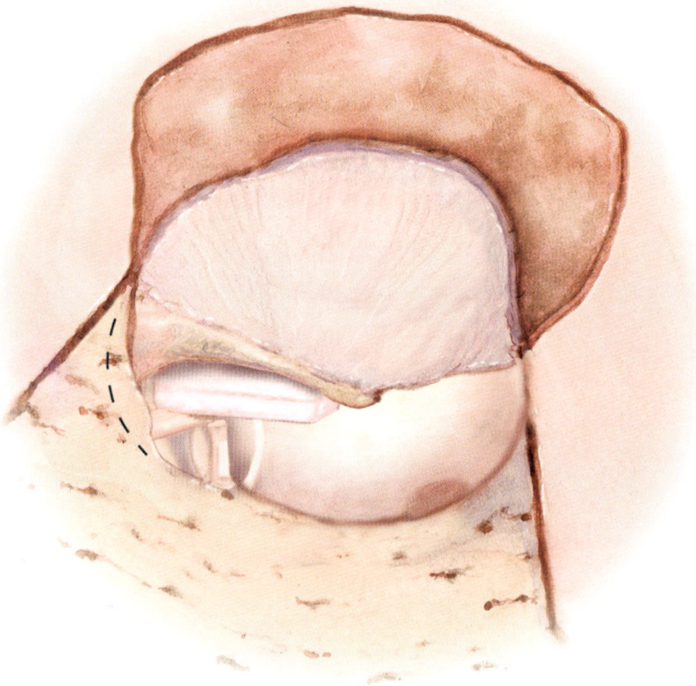

Fig. 5.46

Minor Disruption or Discontinuity of the Incudostapedial Joint

Malleustapedial Interposition

Cartilage can also be placed between the malleus handle and the eroded process of the incus.

Fig. 5.46

Incudostapedial Interposition

In the case of disruption or minor discontinuity (< 2 mm) of the incudostapedial joint, a piece of cartilage can be interposed.

Fig. 5.47

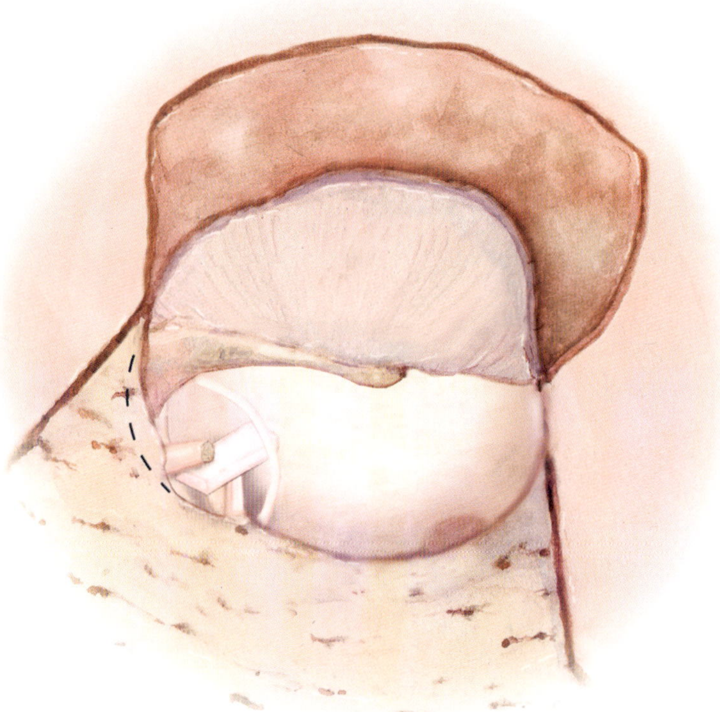

Fig. 5.47

Cement Reconstruction

Biocompatible cement can be placed between the long process of the incus and the head of the stapes.

Fig. 5.48

Tip: A biocompatible cement can be in contact with the tympanic membrane.

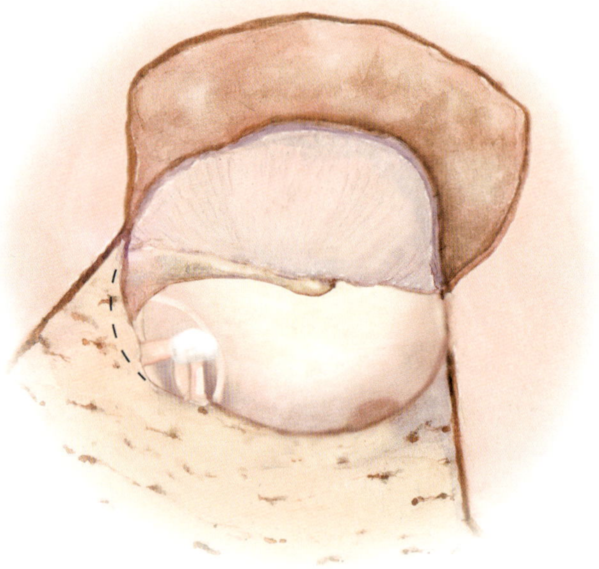

Fig. 5.48

Major Discontinuity of the Incudostapedial Joint (Stapes Useful)

Our preference for type 2 tympanoplasty is autologous incus interposition, if the incus is present, usable, and has no contact with the cholesteatoma membrane. If interposition cannot be considered, titanium prostheses are used.

Removal of the Incus

Before touching the incus, the anatomy of the facial nerve should be visualized and checked. In some cases, it is necessary to perform an atticotomy (see Posterior Epitympanotomy, p. 117).

Incus Mobilization

First, the incus is lateralized, then it is slowly pulled posteriorly using a small hook.

Fig. 5.49

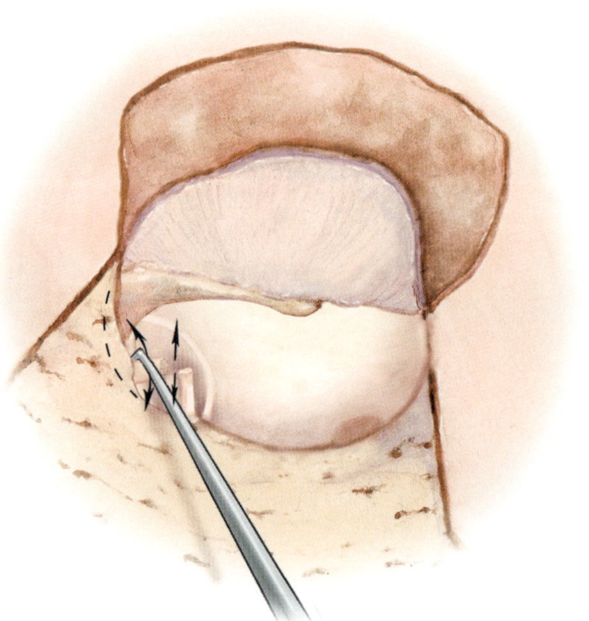

Fig. 5.49

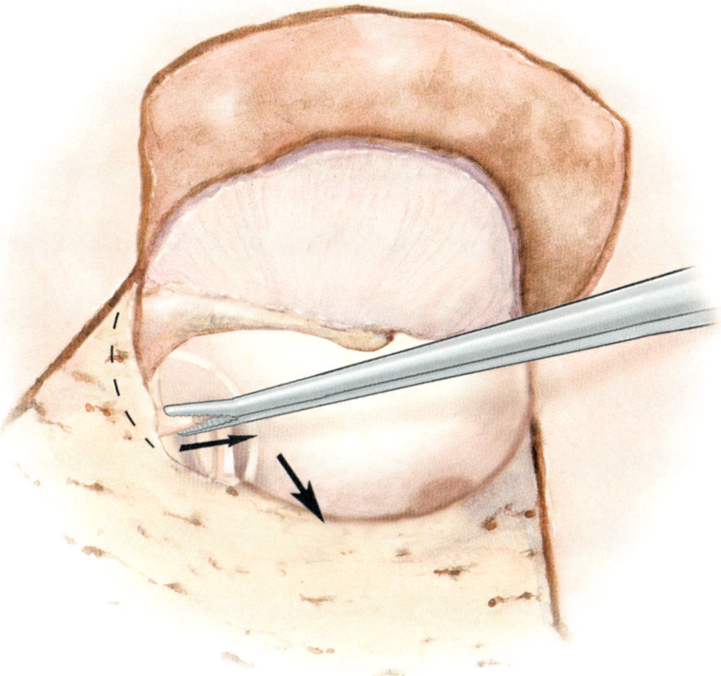

Fig. 5.50

Incus Liberation

The long process of the incus is then grasped with microforceps. Small anteroposterior movements allow the incudomallear joint to be completely liberated before the incus is pulled down and removed.

Fig. 5.50

Tip: Good liberation of the incudomallear joint avoids damage to the long process of the incus with strong movements of the microforceps.
If disarticulation is impossible, a small atticotomy should be performed to visualize and cut the malleus neck with a malleus nipper.

Checking Malleus and Stapes Mobility

If the malleus is fixed, the malleus neck is cut with the malleus nipper and the malleus head is removed, with or without a small atticotomy. The tendon of the tensor tympani muscle may grip the malleus handle. It can be cut with scissors or stretched with a microhook. The mobility of the stapes is checked with a needle.

Fig. 5.51

Tip: If there is any doubt about the mobility, check the movement of the round window when pushing the stapedial head.

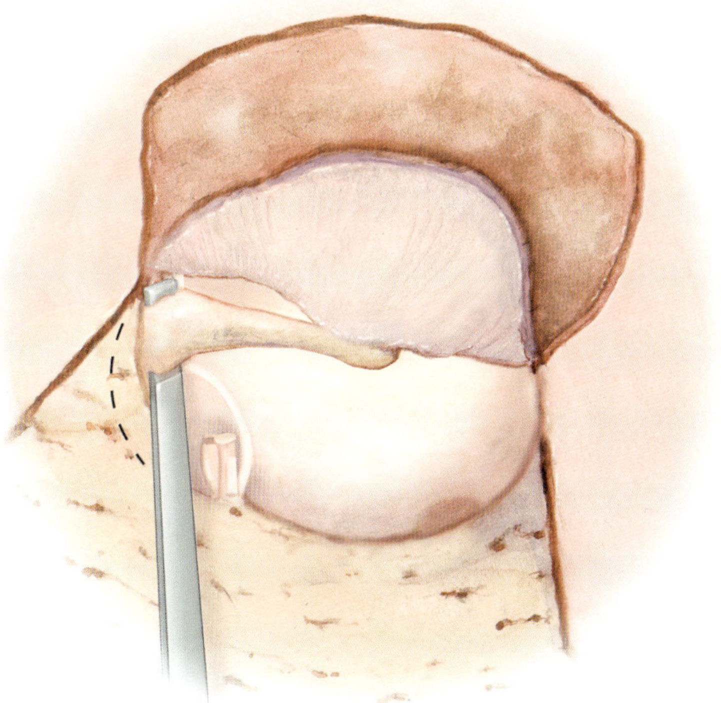

Fig. 5.51

Incus Interposition

Interposition Measurement

Before initiating the procedure of incus shaping, the distance between the head of the stapes and the malleus handle, or the bony annulus if the malleus is absent, should be measured. This can be done with a microinstrument or measuring rod.

Fig. 5.52

Shaping the Incus

The incus body is held with forceps and supported by the left hand (if the surgeon is right-handed). The superior border and articular side are flattened with a diamond burr (A). The long and short process of the incus are drilled and adjusted to the defined size. A small hole is made in its stump using an 0.8-mm diamond burr to hold the stapes head (B).

Fig. 5.53

Tip: If the stapes head is absent, a groove is drilled in the long process stump to fix the interposition over the crura. When the malleus handle is present and suitable, to improve stability, a groove can be made on the superior flattened border of the short process using the same burr.

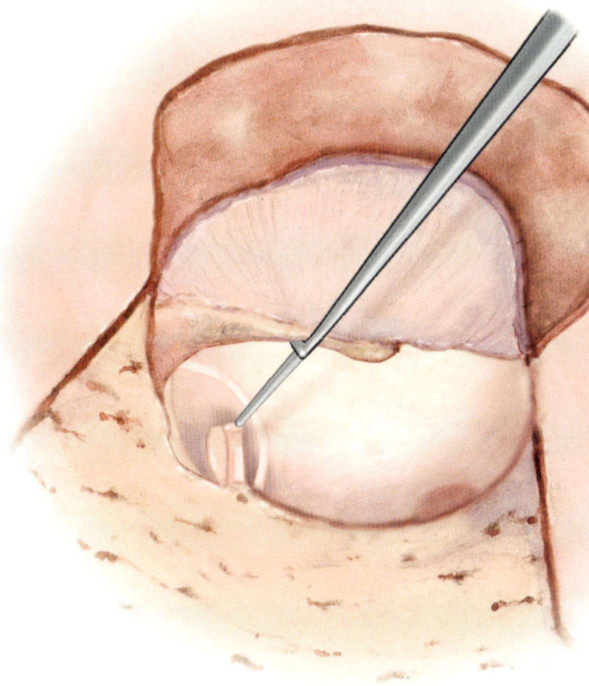

Fig. 5.52

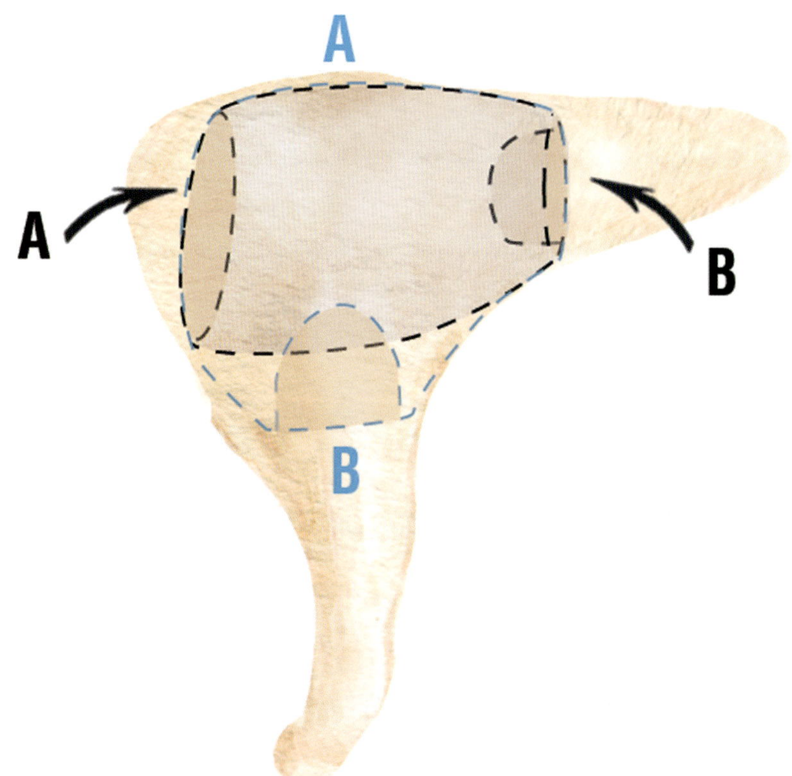

Fig. 5.53

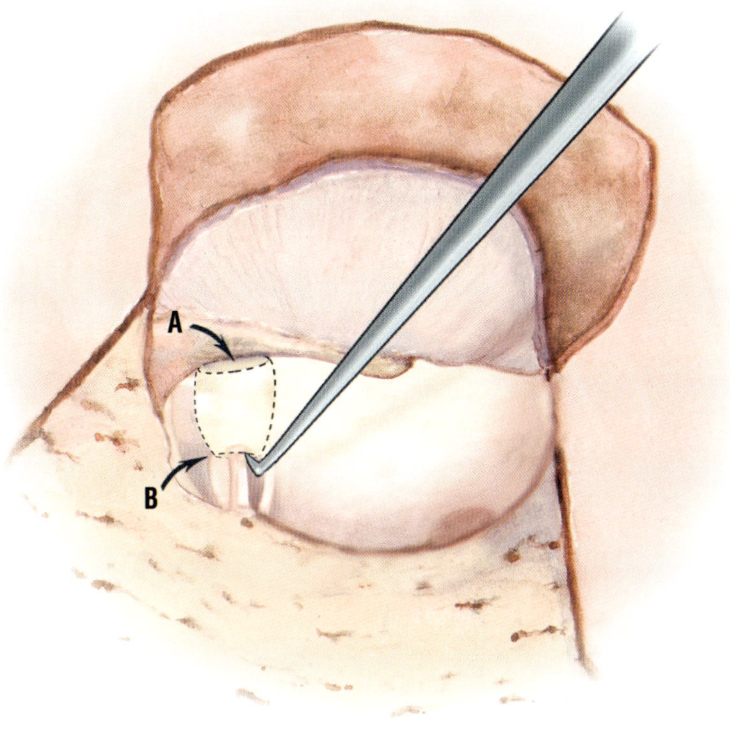

Fig. 5.54

Positioning the Incus (Malleus Handle Present)

Before attempting incus positioning, the tympanic membrane reconstruction should be performed.

The shaped incus is maneuvered into the middle ear cavity by microsuction applied to its head (A). The hole (B) created in the molded incus is then positioned on the stapes head using a microhook.

Fig. 5.54

Positioning the Grooved Incus (Malleus Handle Present)

If the malleus handle is suitable for use and a groove has been created for incus interposition, the malleus is pulled laterally with the microhook and, using a needle, the incus is twisted under the malleus handle.

Fig. 5.55

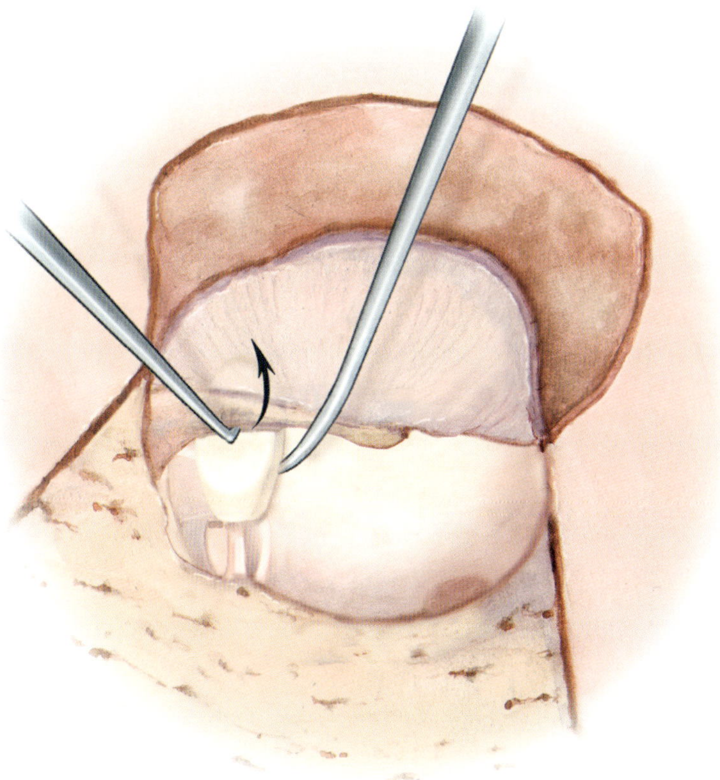

Fig. 5.55

Positioning the Incus (Malleus not Suitable)

If the malleus handle is too retracted and not suitable, the incus interposition is moved into contact with the malleus handle close to its short process. Fibrin glue is added to achieve stability.

Fig. 5.56

Tip: The malleus handle should be used whenever possible. Be careful not to touch the bony annulus with the incus. Spongostan is placed between the incus and the posterior wall to avoid fixation. Do not elevate the malleus handle too far from its initial position, as the tension will block the mobility of the ossiculoplasty. Use the smallest suction diameter to ensure the lowest possible sucking resistance. It helps to disconnect the prosthesis from the suction.

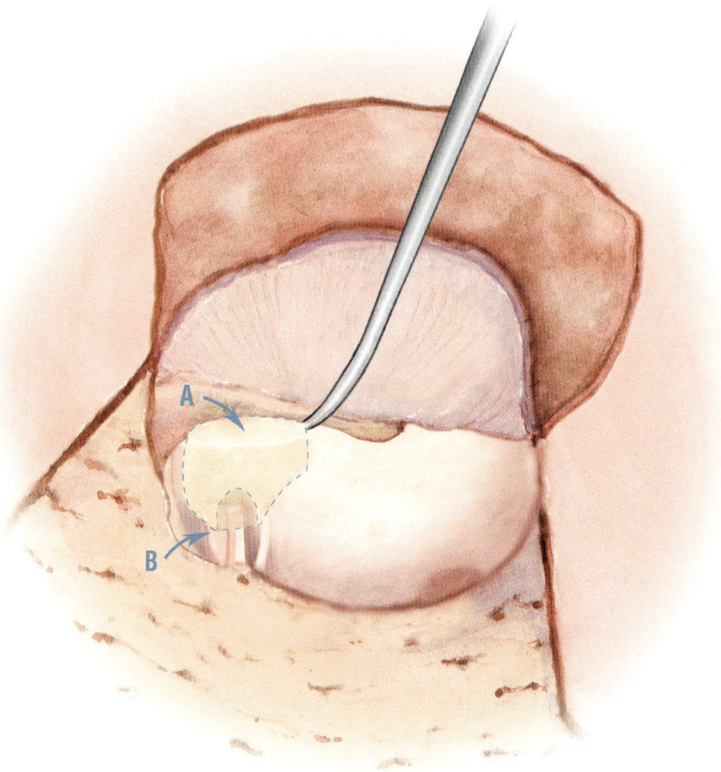

Fig. 5.56

Positioning the Incus (Malleus Handle Absent)

If the malleus is missing, the incus interposition length should be increased. If the columella is too short, cartilage is placed between the columella and the tympanic membrane (A). In the case of tympanic membrane retraction or atticotomy, cartilage interposition of the posterosuperior quadrant is performed, with its perichondrium draping the bony wall.

Fig. 5.57

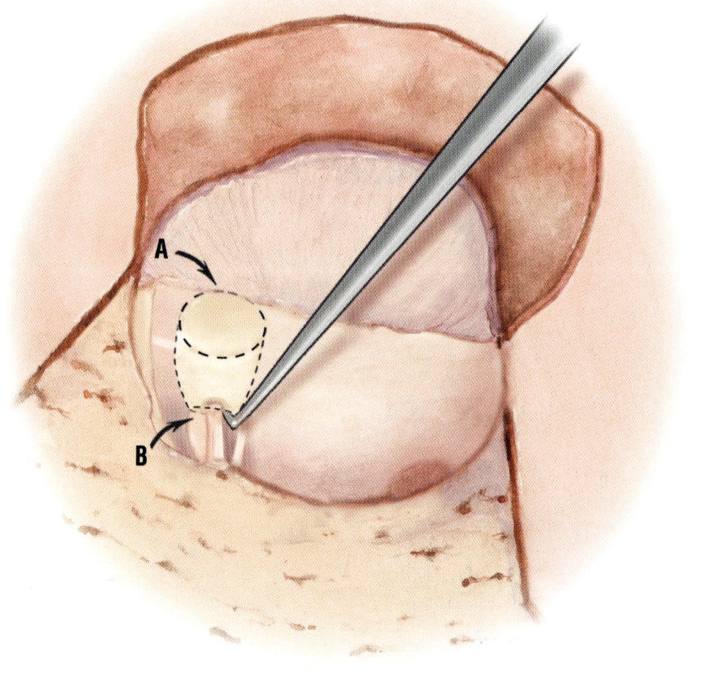

Fig. 5.57

Biocompatible Prostheses

Since 1996 we have used titanium prostheses. We started with those made by Spiggle and Theis GmbH (Overath, Germany) and changed to Kurz 7 years ago.

Our series shows a 3.5% extrusion rate. In all cases the extrusion occurred after interposition of costal cartilage allograft. To avoid this complication, we decided to always use tragal or conchal cartilage for interposition. We use titanium prostheses for their biocompatibility and ease of handling, sizing, and shaping. A titanium prosthesis enhances the intraoperative field of vision, the weight balance facilitates placement, the prosthesis position can be adapted by simple bending, and the prosthesis bell can be crimped onto the stapes head.

Measuring the Prosthesis

The distance between the head of the stapes and the inferior level of the proximal malleus handle, or the bony annulus if the malleus is absent, should be measured using a measuring rod.

Fig. 5.58

Tip: Do not forget that cartilage will be interposed. The cartilage thickness needs to be taken into consideration.

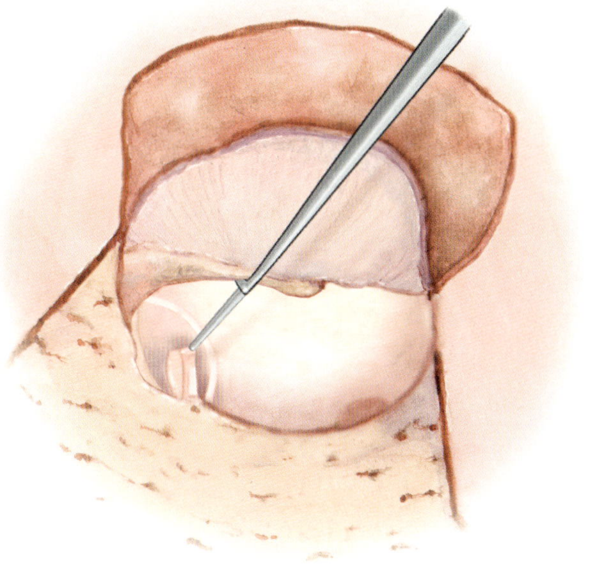

Fig. 5.58

Trying for Size

When the size has been estimated, a specific model from a metal sizer kit should be used (Kurz Middle Ear Implant Sizer Set). Single-use plastic sizer kits are also available (Kurz ACsizer System). The model prosthesis is positioned on the head of the stapes with microsuction pulling its tip and a microhook.

Fig. 5.59

Tip: Establishing the right size and position of the prosthesis improves prosthesis stability and functional results.

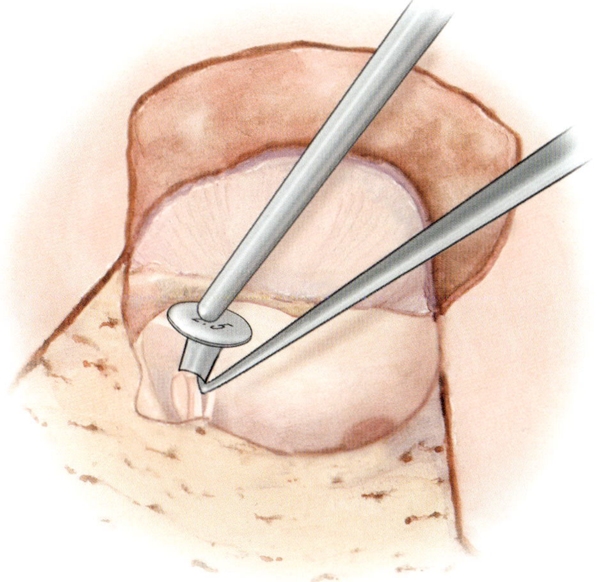

Fig. 5.59

Positioning the Titanium Prosthesis (Malleus Handle Present)

When the perfect size is has been determined, an adjustable prosthesis is prepared and sized, or a presized prosthesis is chosen. The prosthesis is introduced into the middle ear cavity with microsuction applied to the center of the prosthesis plate.

The prosthesis bell is positioned on the stapes head using a needle or microhook (1) and then under the malleus handle (2).

Fig. 5.60

Positioning the Titanium Prosthesis under the Malleus Handle

If the malleus handle is suitable, the malleus is pulled laterally using a microhook and a needle is used to twist the prothesis under the malleus handle. If the malleus handle is too retracted and not suitable, the prosthesis is moved into contact with the malleus handle close to its short process. To achieve stability, fibrin glue is added to the ossiculoplasty.

Fig. 5.61

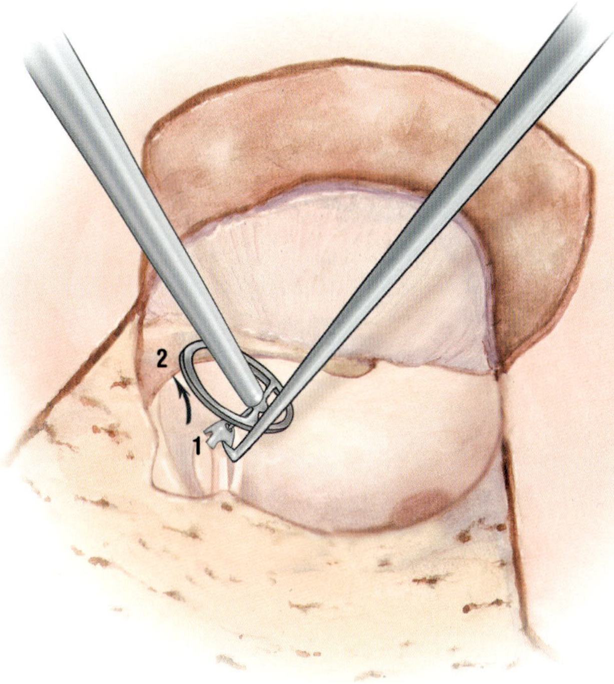

Fig. 5.60

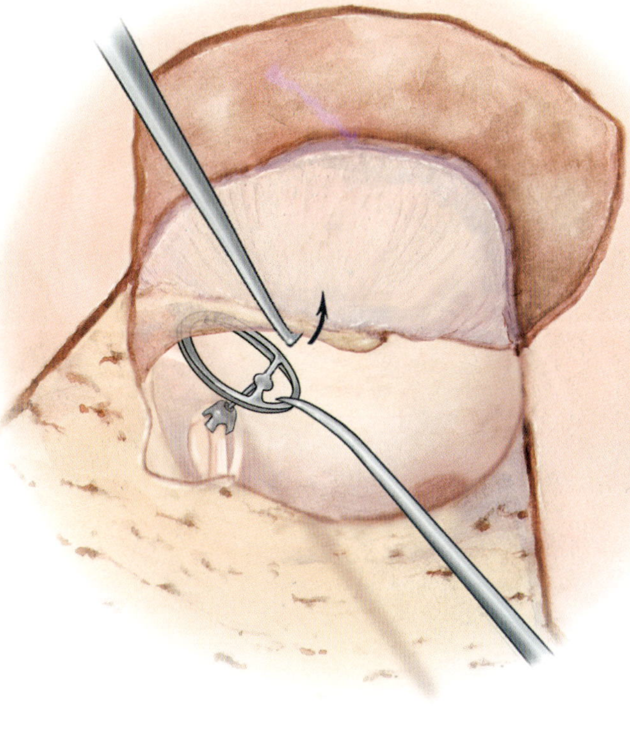

Fig. 5.61

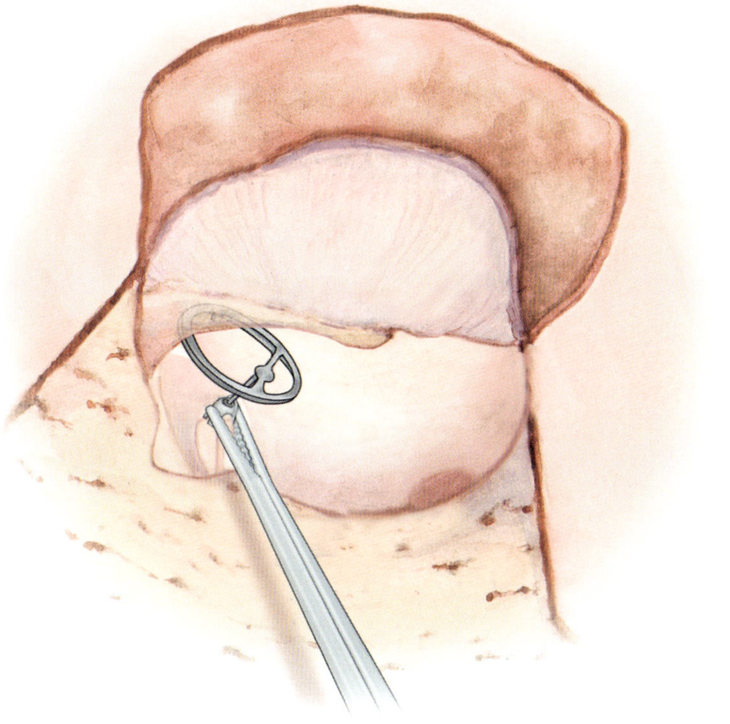

Fig. 5.62

Crimping the Prosthesis Bell
To improve stability and sound conduction, it is a good idea to crimp the prosthesis bell onto the stapes head using microforceps.
Fig. 5.62

Tip: Crimping improves prosthesis stability. This step is more important if the malleus is absent or if the prosthesis plate is not positioned beneath the malleus handle. Do not crimp too firmly, however, or it may be difficult and dangerous to remove the prosthesis during revision surgery.

Cartilage Interposition
Cartilage is always interposed with titanium prostheses.

Tragal or conchal cartilage chips should cover the prosthesis plate, but not the bony annulus.
Fig. 5.63

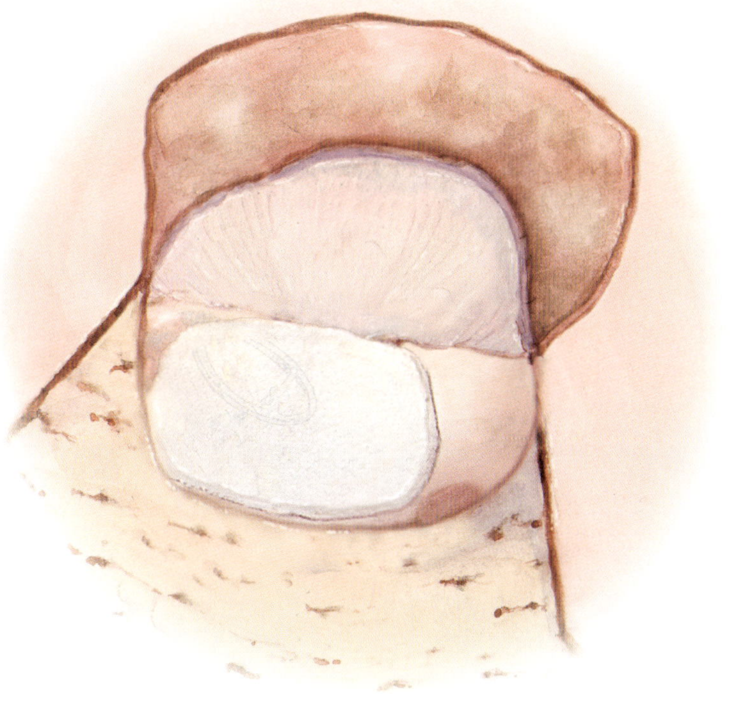

Fig. 5.63

Cartilage–Perichondrium Interposition

In the case of tympanic membrane retraction or atticotomy, a larger cartilage interposition to cover the posterosuperior quadrant is performed, with its perichondrium draping the bony wall (see Management of Controlled Posterior or Posterior Attic Retraction Pockets, p. 110).

Fig. 5.64

Tip: Do not hesitate to use a palisade of small cartilage chips. To reduce extrusion, we recommend covering the posterosuperior quadrant with interposed cartilage, avoiding gaps between the bony annulus and the cartilage chips. Be careful not to touch the bony annulus with the incus. Spongostan is placed between the incus and the posterior wall to avoid fixation. Do not elevate the malleus handle too far from its initial position as the tension will block the mobility of the ossiculoplasty. Use the smallest suction diameter to ensure the lowest possible sucking resistance. It helps to disconnect the prosthesis from the suction.

Positioning the Titanium Prosthesis (Malleus Handle Absent)

In this case, the prosthesis length should be measured between the stapes head and the bony annulus. Prosthesis stability is very important and can be enhanced through bell crimping, tympanic reconstruction, and cartilage interposition.

Fig. 5.65

Tip: We believe that using small cartilage chips is an excellent way to preserve the three-dimensional anatomy of the eardrum and improve the stability of the ossiculoplasty.

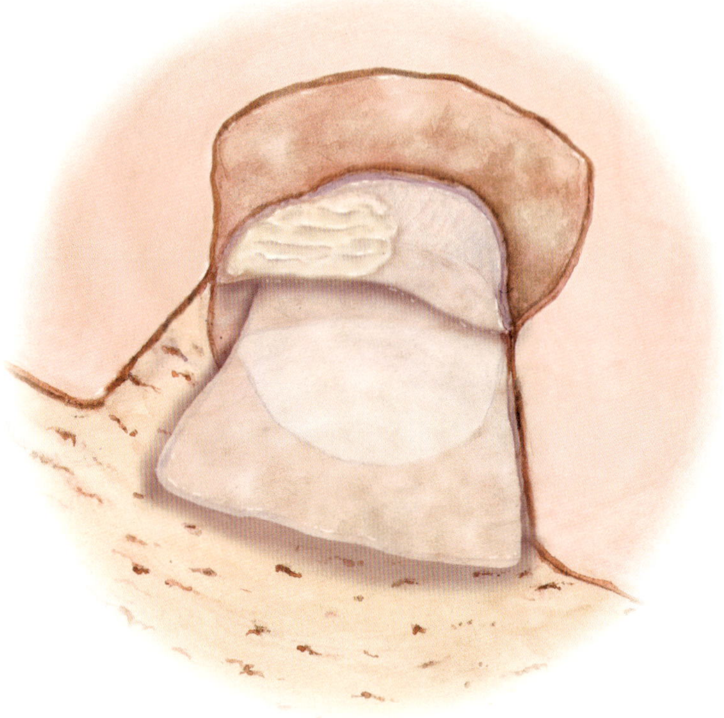

Fig. 5.64

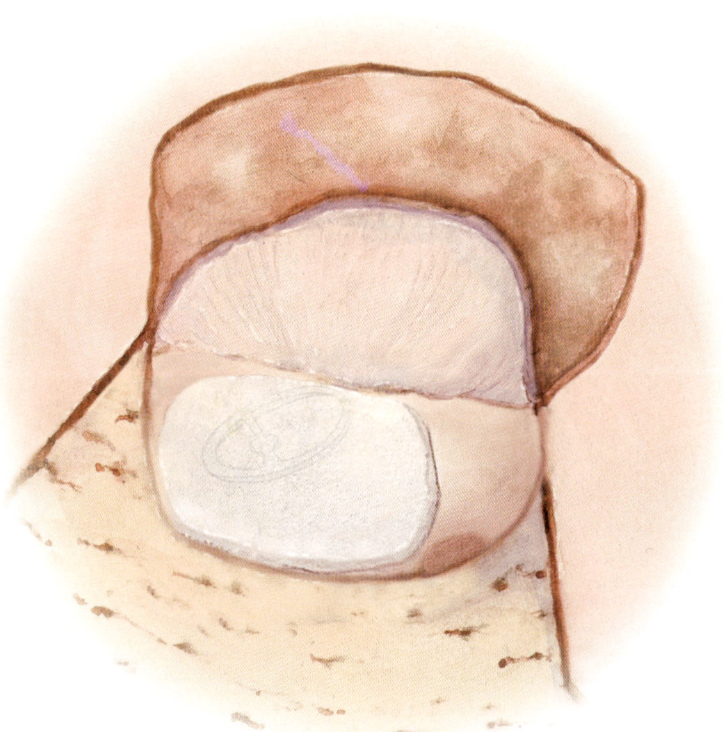

Fig. 5.65

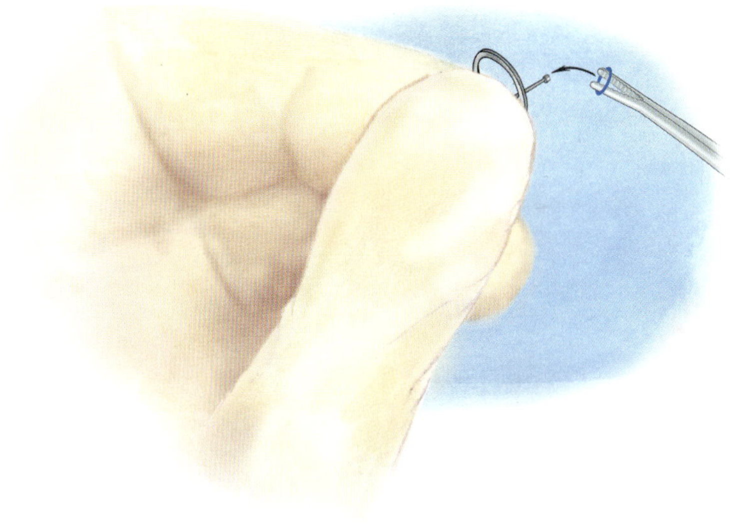

Fig. 5.66

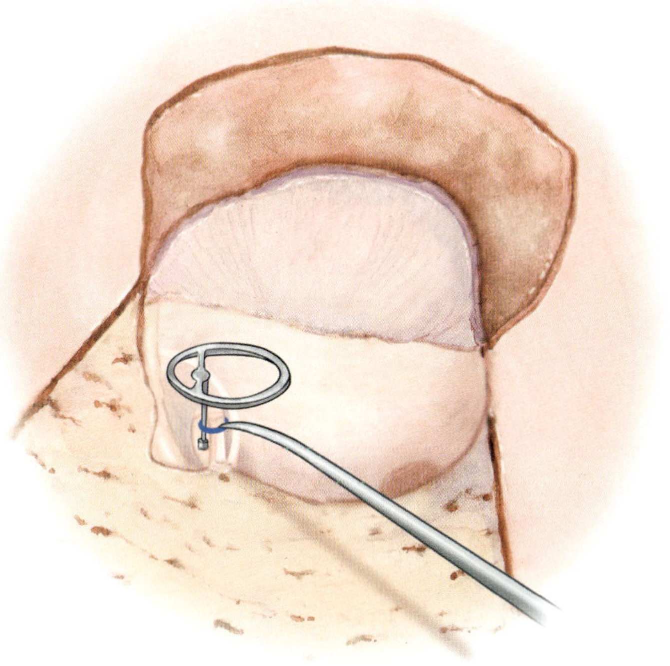

Fig. 5.67

Silastic Banding

The Silastic banding technique was described by R. Vincent of the J. B. Causse Ear Clinic (Vincent et al. 2005). To create a Silastic ring, a small disk is cut from a thin Silastic sheet using a 2-mm-diameter Lempert suction tube on a metallic sheet. A hole is made in the Silastic disk center using 0.8-mm-diameter microsuction.

Silastic Banding, Placement

The Silastic ring is placed around the prosthesis shaft using microforceps.

Fig. 5.66

Silastic Banding, Positioning

The whole prosthesis is positioned on the footplate without removing the superstructure. The Silastic ring is stretched with a needle and attached to the stapes head.

Fig. 5.67

Tip: Attach the banding to the stapes head first and then adjust the prosthesis position. In the case of a partially destroyed head, a small piece of temporalis fascia placed around the banding and destroyed head may improve stability. This technique can be used both with a normal superstructure and if the malleus is absent.

When the malleus handle is absent or too retracted, Silastic banding can also be considered. This technique may allow better stability than a type 2 ossiculoplasty.

Fig. 5.68, Fig. 5.69

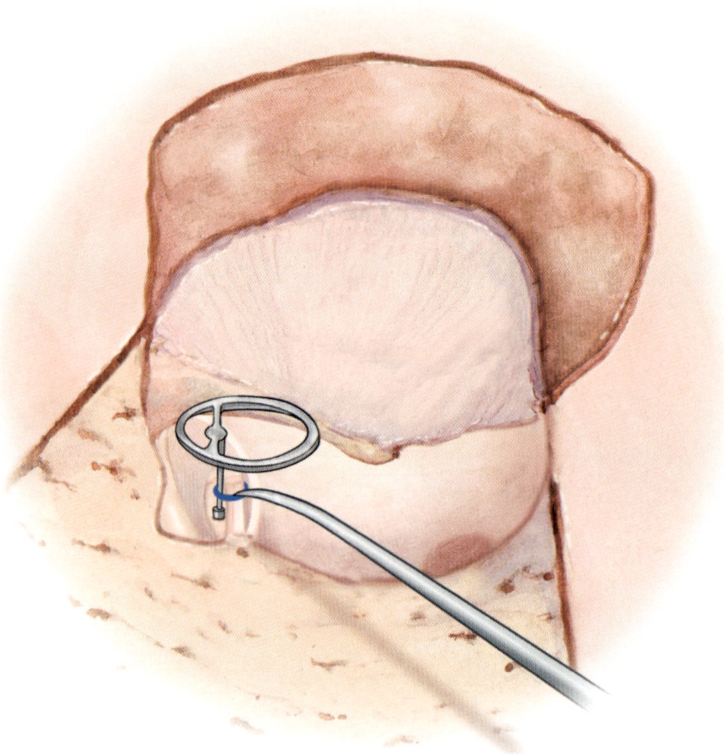

Fig. 5.68

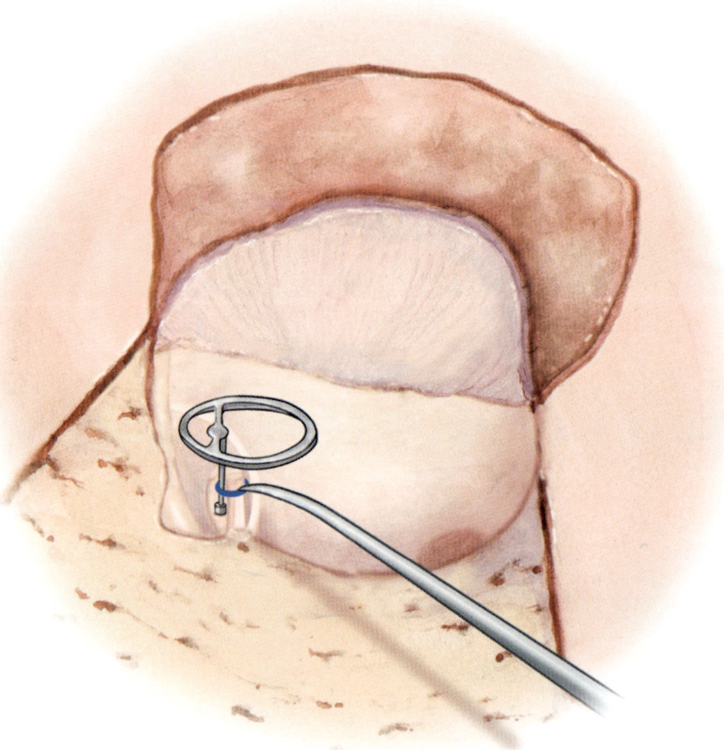

Fig. 5.69

Major Discontinuity of the Incudostapedial Joint (Redundant Stapes Superstructure)

Useless Stapes

In rare cases, the stapes superstructure has a partially destroyed capitulum or the stapes is tilted toward the promontory, and a type 2 ossiculoplasty may be too difficult to attempt. The silastic banding technique should be considered.
Fig. 5.70

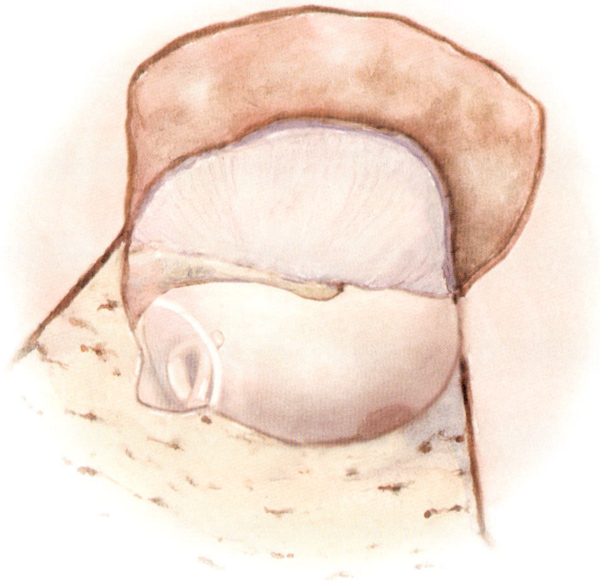

Fig. 5.70

If the stapes superstructure is absent, removed, partially destroyed, or tilted, a titanium total ossicular replacement prosthesis (TORP) is used for ossiculoplasty. Biocompatible prostheses are preferred, since in our opinion they yield better functional and stability results than incus or malleus interposition. Footplate mobility must first be checked using a needle.

Missing Stapes Superstructure

Prosthesis Measurement

The distance between the footplate and the inferior level of the proximal malleus handle, or bony annulus if the malleus is absent, is measured with a measuring rod.
Fig. 5.71

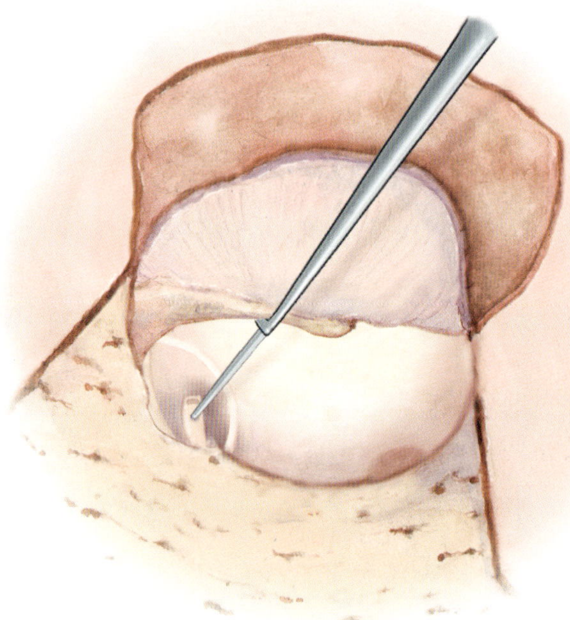

Fig. 5.71

Total Ossiculoplasty (Malleus Present)

The prosthesis is introduced into the middle ear cavity using microsuction applied to the center of the prosthesis plate. The prosthesis is positioned on the footplate with a needle or microhook. If the malleus handle is suitable for use, the malleus is pulled laterally with the microhook, and a needle is used to twist the prosthesis plate under the proximal malleus handle. If the malleus handle is too retracted and not suitable, the prosthesis is moved into contact with the malleus handle close to its short process. To achieve stability, fibrin glue is added to the ossiculoplasty. Cartilage interposition is always performed (see Cartilage Interposition, p. 98).

Fig. 5.72

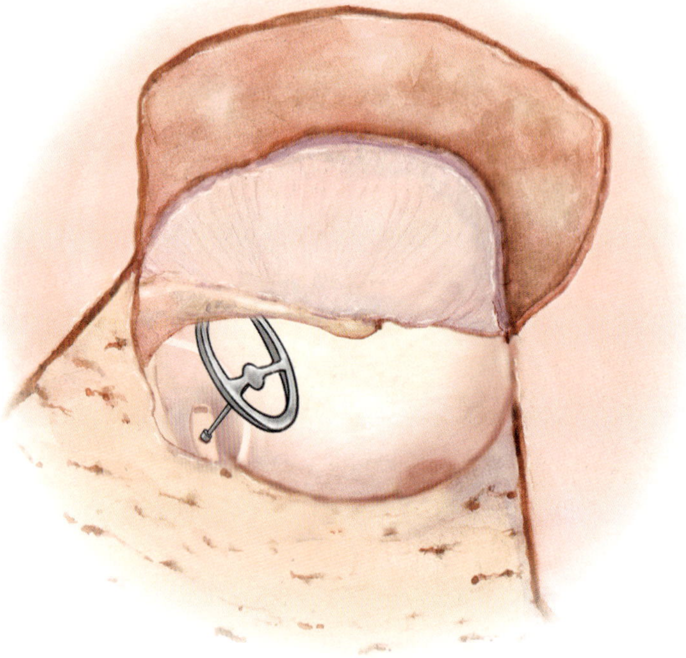

Fig. 5.72

Tip: Very small Spongostan pieces or, even better, cartilage chips can be placed around the footplate to improve prosthesis stability. The prosthesis should be positioned as perpendicularly as possible to the footplate.

Total Ossiculoplasty (Malleus Absent)

In this case, we perform cartilage interposition on the footplate to optimize prosthesis stability and position.

Preparation of Footplate–Cartilage Interposition

Using a Hüttenbrink cartilage punch (Kurz), a small cartilage plate is created from tragal or conchal cartilage chips. It corresponds to the size of the oval niche and is perforated in its center to hold the prosthesis foot.

Fig. 5.73

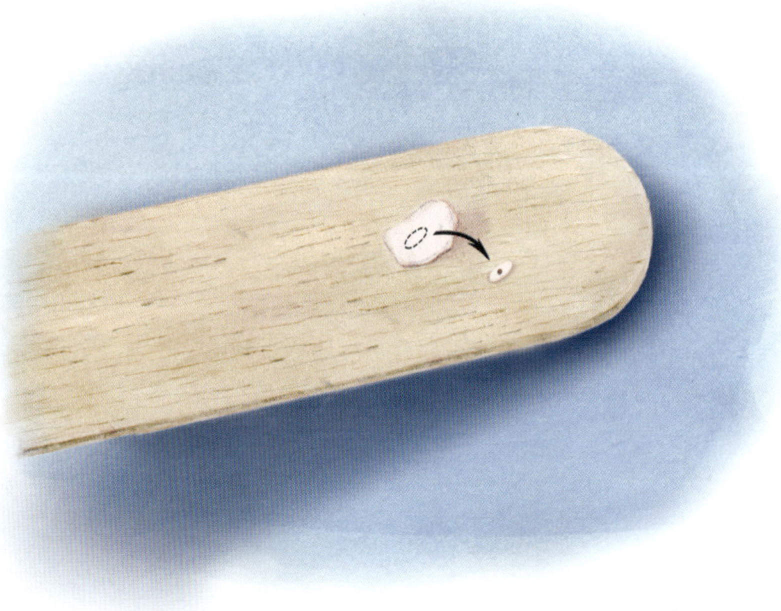

Fig. 5.73

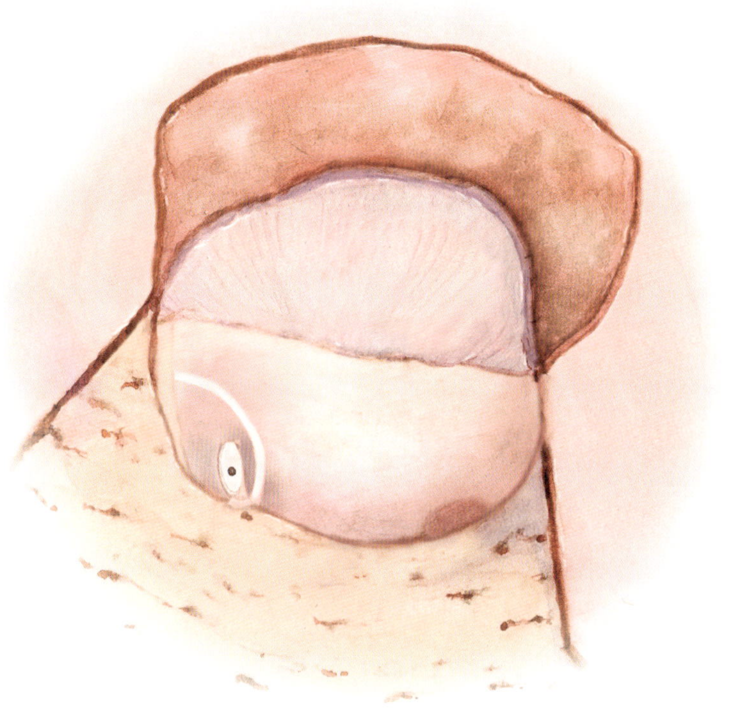

Fig. 5.74

Positioning the Footplate–Cartilage Interposition

The cartilage interposition is placed on the footplate using a needle. If the cartilage does not fit the footplate in size, it can be reshaped. The prosthesis foot is inserted into the cartilage perforation with a needle or microhook and the cartilage plate is stabilized using gentle microsuction.

Fig. 5.74

Positioning the Prosthesis in the Footplate–Cartilage Interposition

The prosthesis is moved into position using the needle.

Fig. 5.75

Tip: Very small Spongostan pieces or, even better, cartilage chips can be placed around the footplate to improve prosthesis stability. Be careful not to touch the bony annulus or facial nerve with the prosthesis. To avoid contact with the bony annulus, do not hesitate to enlarge the posterior epitympanotomy. The shaft can be bent to avoid facial canal contact. Spongostan can be placed to avoid fixation of the prosthesis plate, to the bony annulus. Use the smallest suction diameter to ensure the lowest possible sucking resistance. It helps to disconnect the prosthesis from the suction.

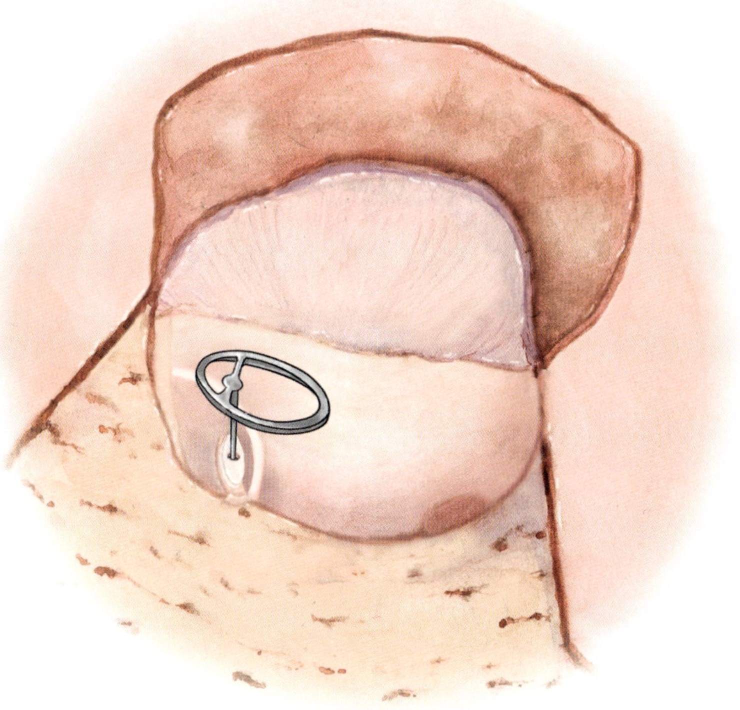

Fig. 5.75

6

Management of Retraction Pockets and Cholesteatoma

6__Management of Retraction Pockets and Cholesteatoma

The different classifications of retraction pockets and cholesteatomas are directly related to the different dysfunctions of middle ear ventilation pathways (see Middle Ear Ventilation, p. 4).

Classification of Retraction Pockets (according to Gersdorff)

Noncholesteatomatous retraction pockets:

Type 1: Mobile, reversible upon ventilation
Type 2 a: Adherent, self-cleaning, wholly visible with a microscope
Type 2 b: Wholly visible with an endoscope only
Type 3: Adherent, self-cleaning, beyond view with either the microscope or the endoscope (= precholesteatoma)

Cholesteatomatous retraction pockets:

Type 4: Adherent, not self-cleaning, with accumulation of keratin, epithelial debris (= cholesteatoma on retraction pocket)
Type 5: Adherent, not self-cleaning, with otorrhea and/or inflammatory granuloma (= infected cholesteatoma)

Classification of Cholesteatomas

Mesotympanic

Protympanic

Retrotympanic

Fig. 6.1

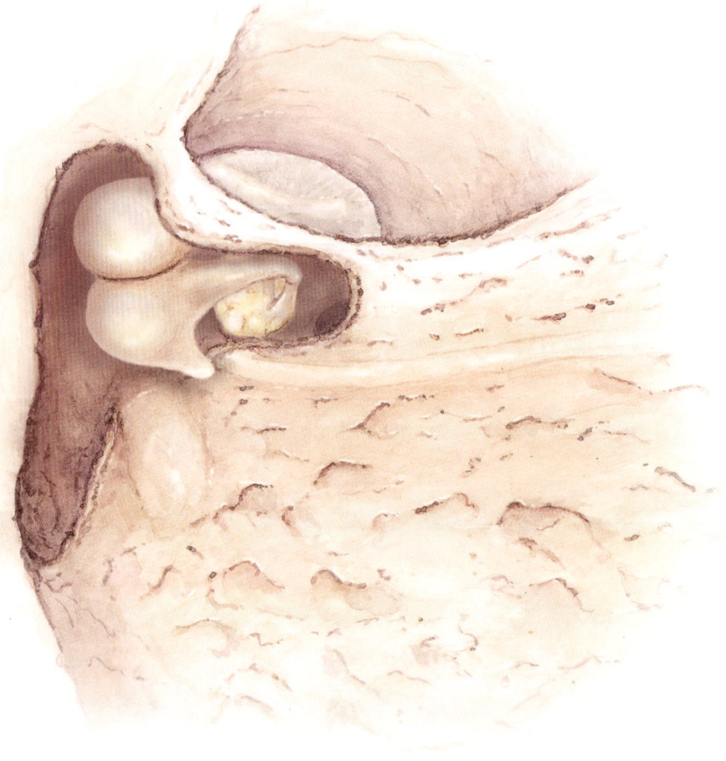

Fig. 6.1

Retrotympanic with Mastoid Extension

Fig. 6.2

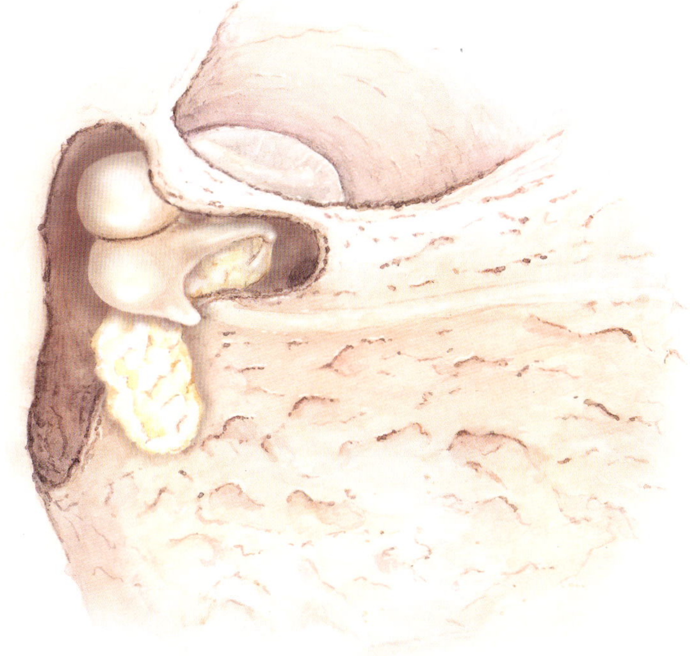

Fig. 6.2

Epitympanic

Anterior Epitympanic

Fig. 6.3

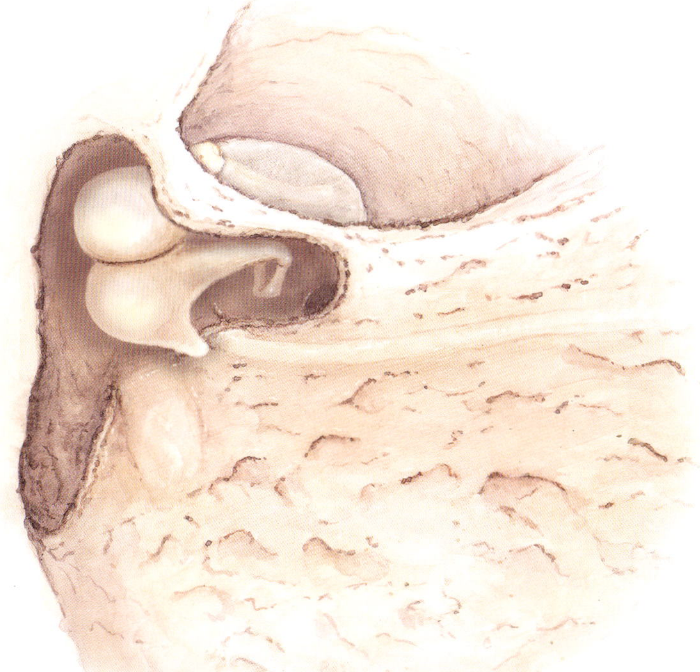

Fig. 6.3

Anterior Epitympanic with Medial Extension (Supratubal Fossa)
Fig. 6.4

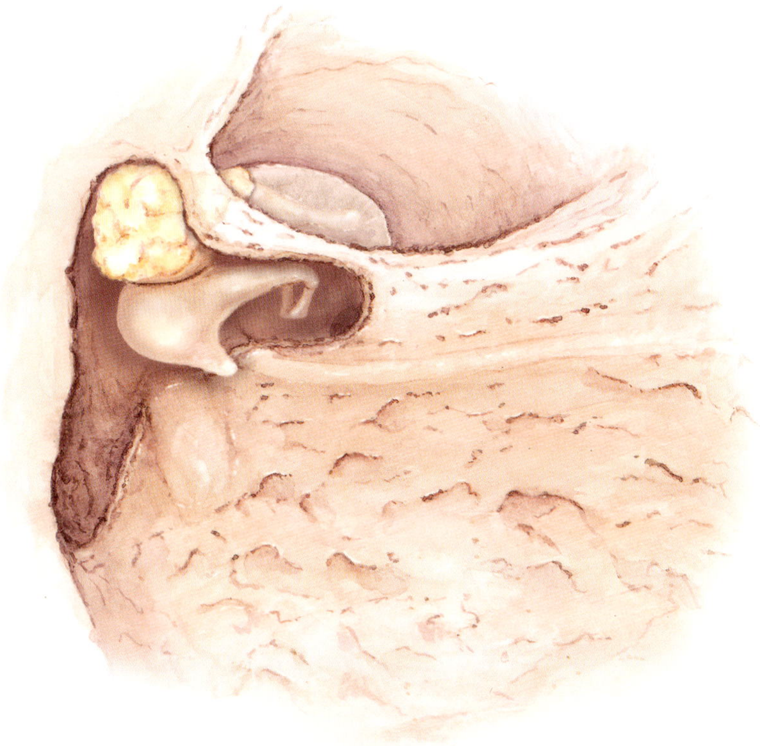

Fig. 6.4

Posterior Epitympanic
Fig. 6.5

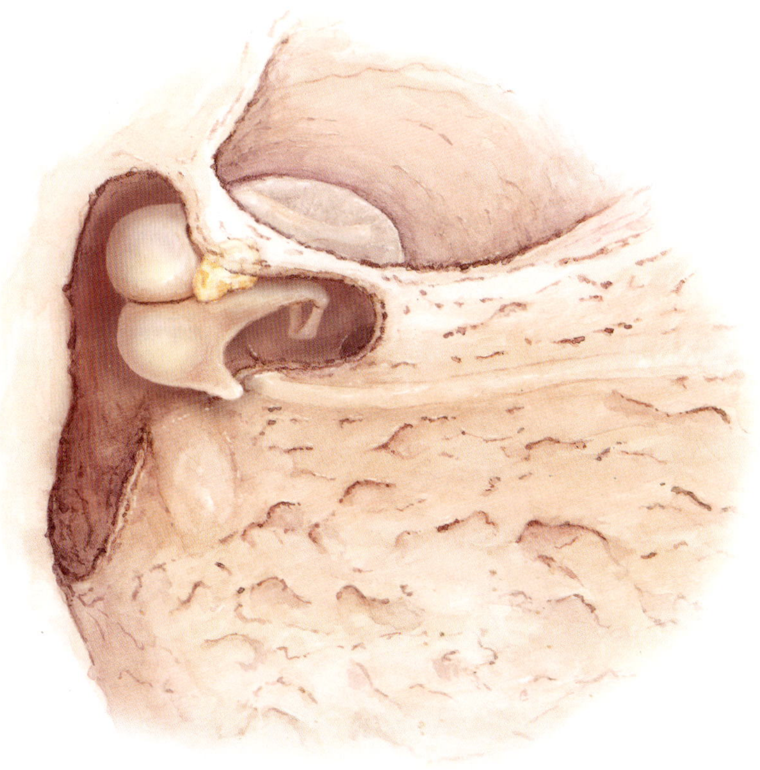

Fig. 6.5

Posterior Epitympanic with Mastoid Extension

Fig. 6.6

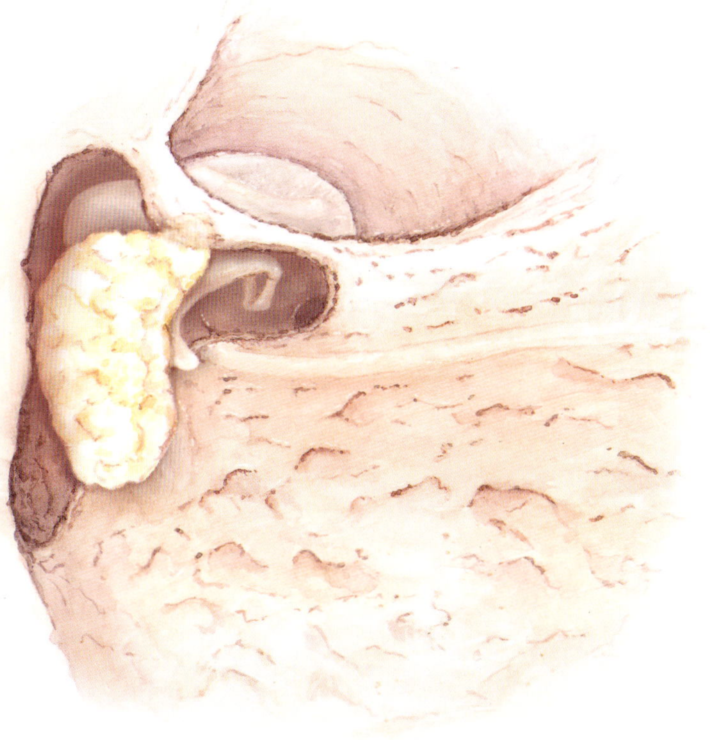

Fig. 6.6

Holotympanic

Holotympanic Starting from Retrotympanum or Posterior Attic with Mastoid Extension

Fig. 6.7

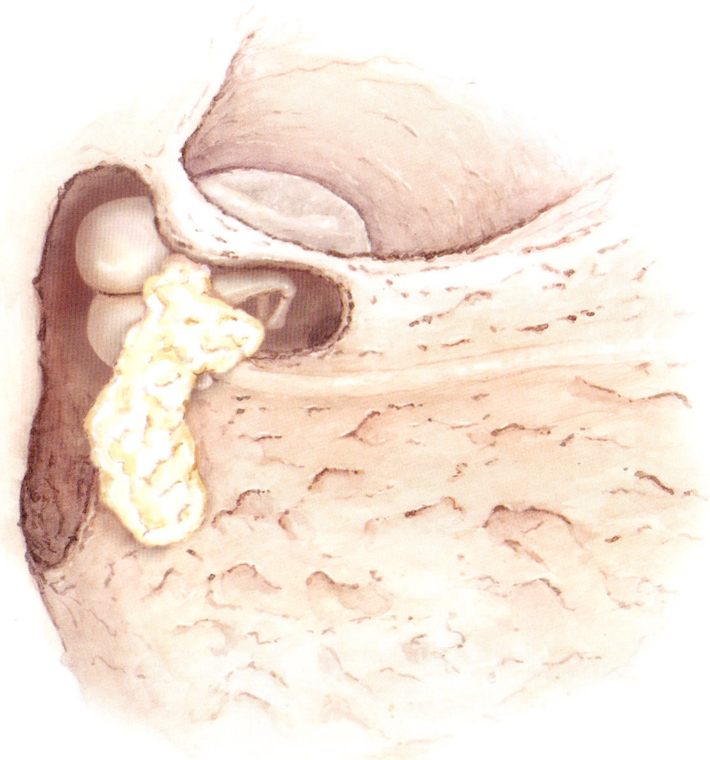

Fig. 6.7

Management Philosophy

Only retraction pockets with no self-cleaning properties and which show recurrent otorrhea and ossicular chain defects leading to significant conductive hearing loss should be operated on.

We perform mastoidectomy only for cholesteatomas of the mastoid cavity and for those originating in the tympanic cavity that cannot be satisfactorily managed by a transmeatal approach, with or without tympanoatticotomy.

In most cases, we use a canal-wall-up (CWU) technique, except in the case of very large defects of the external auditory bony canal wall eroding the mastoid, large recurrent or residual cholesteatomas, or large labyrinthine fistulas, or in patients with large cholesteatomas who are at high risk from anesthesia or regarded as unreliable for follow-up.

We perform one-stage surgery, except in the case of very large and aggressive cholesteatomas, uncontrolled stapes cholesteatomas, infected cholesteatomas, large bony defects, mucosal inflammation, and poor middle ear ventilation.

The CWU technique also requires good-quality imaging follow-up. After cholesteatoma surgery, patients undergo an MRI exam at 12 months. If residual or recurrent cholesteatoma is suspected, a CT scan is performed. In the future, systematic MRI will probably replace the second-look procedure.

Revision surgery is performed in cases of functional failure, residual cholesteatoma suspected on follow-up CT scan or MRI, and recurrent cholesteatoma.

For further follow-up, an MRI exam is performed once a year for 5 years, especially in children.

Management of Controlled Posterior or Posterior Attic Retraction Pockets

Tympanomeatal Flap Incision

For retraction pockets, the meatal skin flap length must be at least 8–10 mm.

A retraction pocket with little epitympanic erosion can be managed using a transmeatal approach, with or without extended tympanoatticotomy.

Fig. 6.8

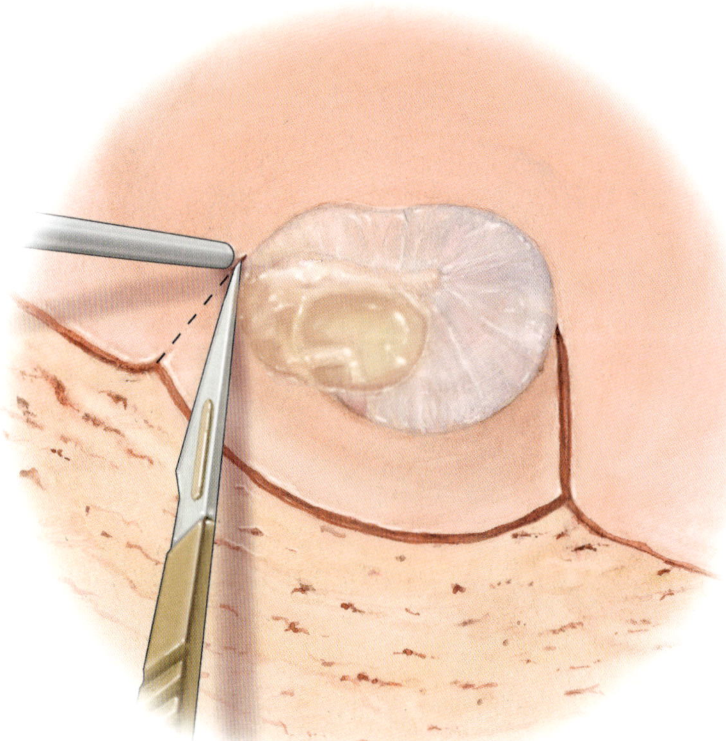

Fig. 6.8

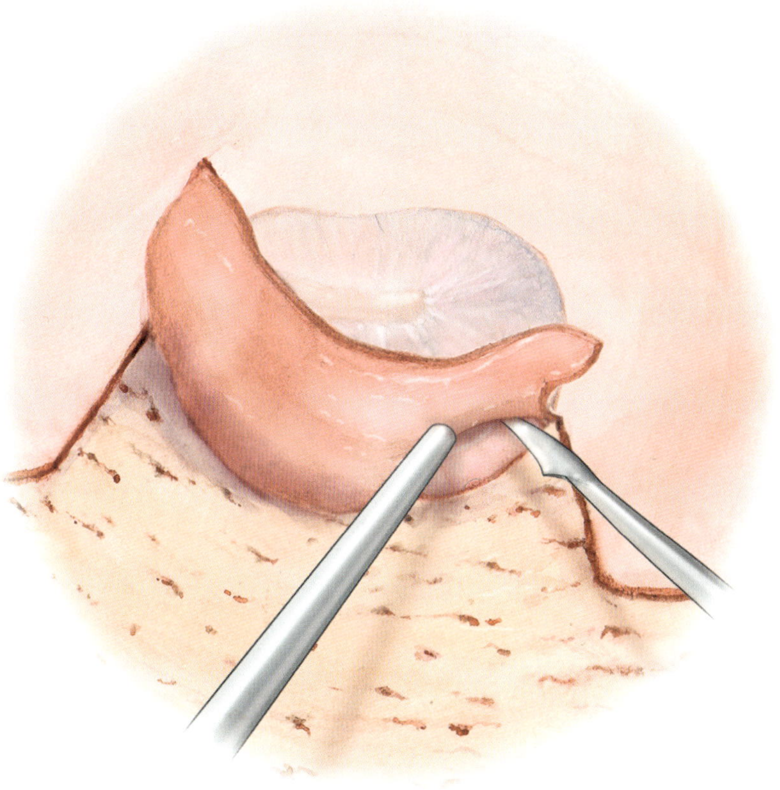

Fig. 6.9

Fibrous Annulus Dislocation

With a needle or sickle knife, the fibrous annulus is dislocated from its sulcus, beginning at the inferior level where the tympanic cavity is aerated.

Fig. 6.9

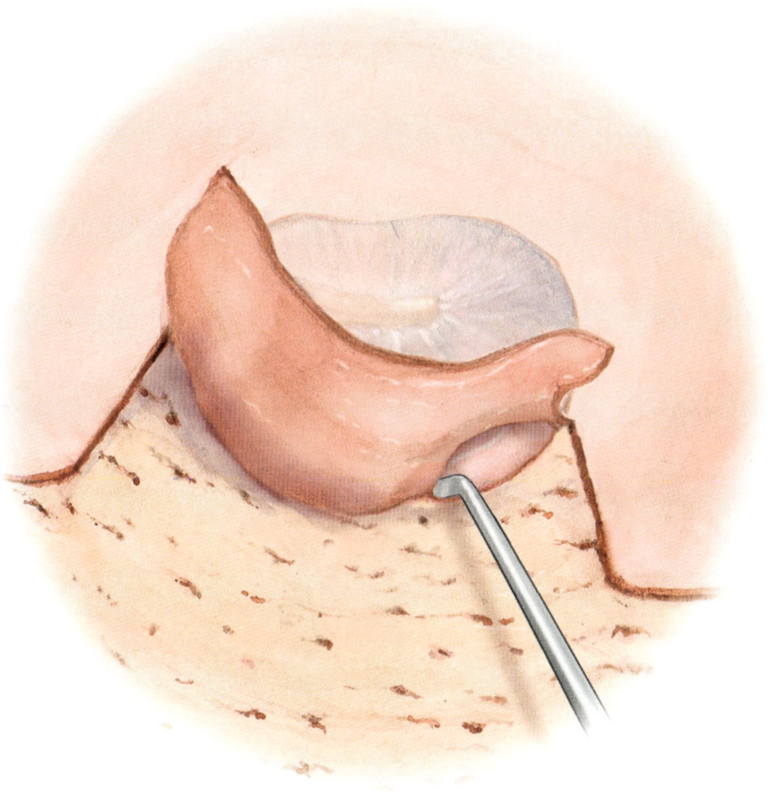

Fig. 6.10

Tympanic Membrane Dislocation

If the opening is large enough, a flap knife or dissector-elevator is inserted and the retraction pocket is slowly dissected and pushed out with the dissector-elevator. Sometimes, it requires use of a longer instrument called a meatus dissector-elevator.

Epidermic dissection of fragile structures, such as the incus, stapes superstructure, footplates, and chorda tympani, is required and should be carefully performed (see Hypotympanic, Protympanic, and Mesotympanic Cholesteatoma, p. 122).

Fig. 6.10

Posterior Tympanoatticotomy

Depending on the extension of the retraction pocket, a posterior tympanoatticotomy is performed with a chisel or curette.

The tympanoatticotomy location allows different tympanic cavity approaches. Posterior tympanoatticotomy is the most common opening technique. It is used for middle ear exploration, ossiculoplasty with intact tympanic membrane, stapes surgery, and management of pathologies of the posterior tympanum

Fig. 6.11

Uncontrolled Extension

In the case of uncontrolled extension of a cholesteatoma to the facial recess and sinus tympani, a posterior tympanotomy is performed (see Posterior Tympanotomy, p. 119).

Fig. 6.12

Tip: Enter the middle ear cavity where the tympanic membrane is not retracted, but aerated, and slowly push out the retraction pocket to prevent tearing. Try to preserve the integrity of the tympanic membrane and also ensure that residual epithelium is not left behind. When the round window niche is recognized, proceed down to the pyramid and oval window. This can be checked using Zini mirrors or specially adapted otoendoscopes. If in doubt, perform a mastoid approach. Posterior tympanoatticotomy can also be extended to anterior tympanoatticotomy and/or inferior tympanotomy, if there is any pathological extension. If a drill is used for the tympanoatticotomy, remove the final bony overhang with a curette to avoid ossicular chain damage.

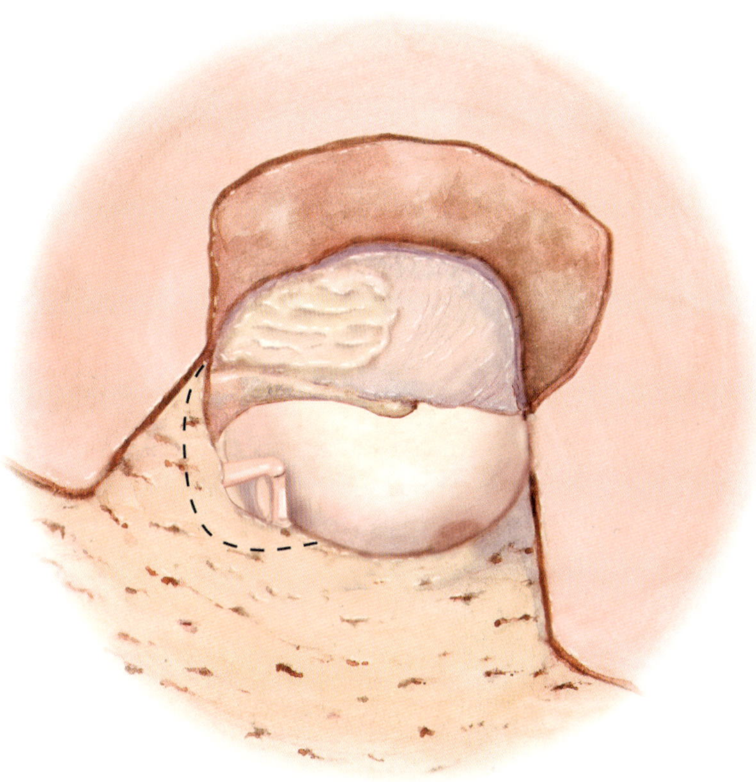

Fig. 6.11

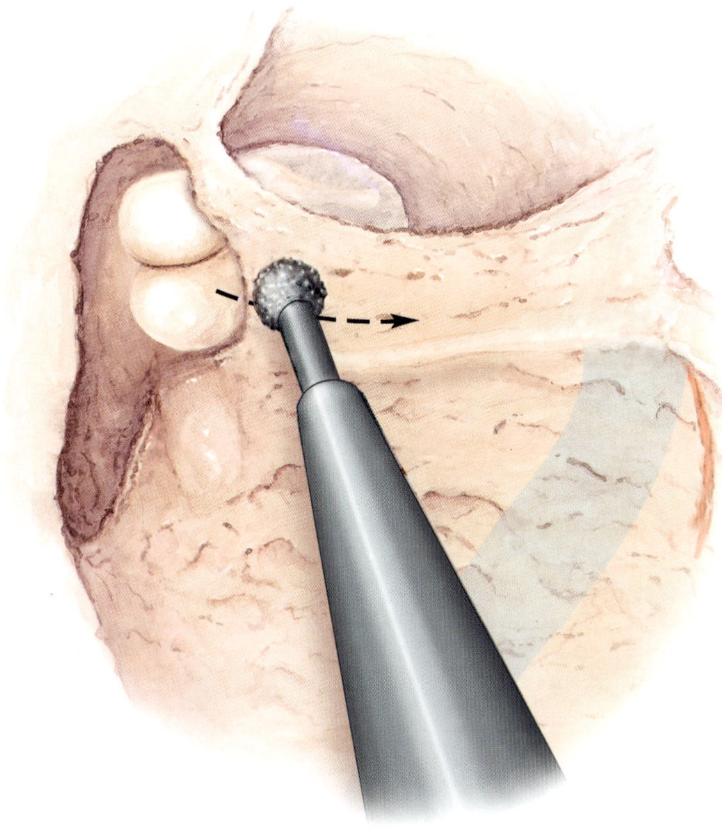

Fig. 6.12

Cartilage–Perichondium Graft

The tympanic membrane is repaired using a tragal cartilage–perichondrium graft covering at least the posterior quadrants, the retracted tympanic membrane surface, and the bony wall defect (see Cartilage Tympanoplasty, p. 61).

Fig. 6.13

Tip: Do not forget to check the integrity of the ossicular chain and repair it if necessary.

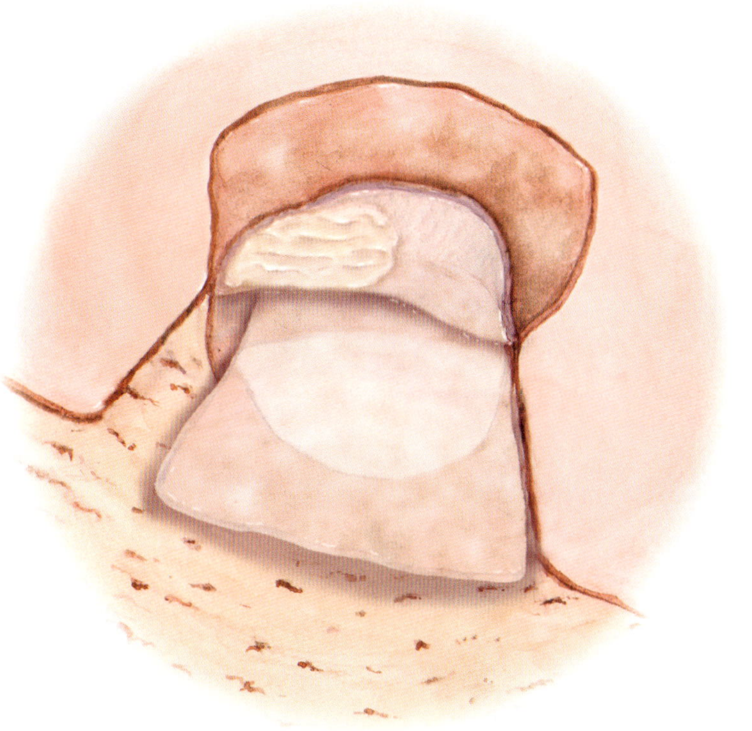

Fig. 6.13

Management of Controlled Anterior Attic Retraction Pockets

Tympanomeatal Incision

The superior lateral skin incision is extended to the anterior canal wall several millimeters above the retraction pocket border. An anterior tympanoatticotomy is performed through a transmeatal approach using a small curette.

Fig. 6.14

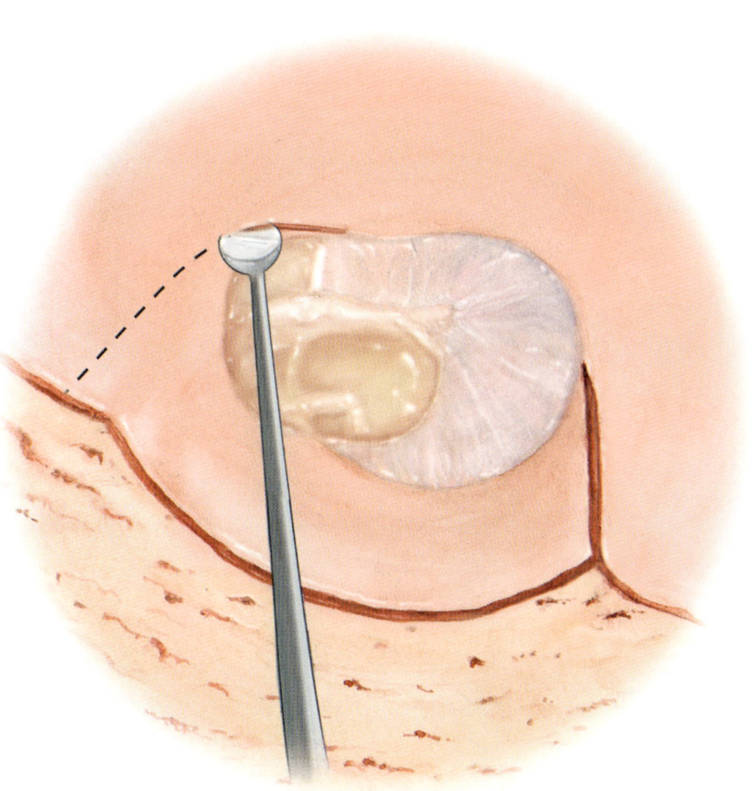

Fig. 6.14

Posterior Epitympanotomy

If there is any doubt regarding the presence of epithelium on the malleus head or cholesteatoma in the anterior epitympanum, a posterior epitympanotomy should be performed through a mastoidectomy (see Posterior Epitympanotomy, p. 117).

Fig. 6.15

The incus is removed and the malleus head cut. The cog (bony crest between the anterior and posterior epitympanum) is then removed using a diamond burr to open the anterior epitympanum and clean it.

The retraction pocket is pushed out from the epitympanic area to the external auditory canal using the dissector-elevator with or without a soaked cotton ball.

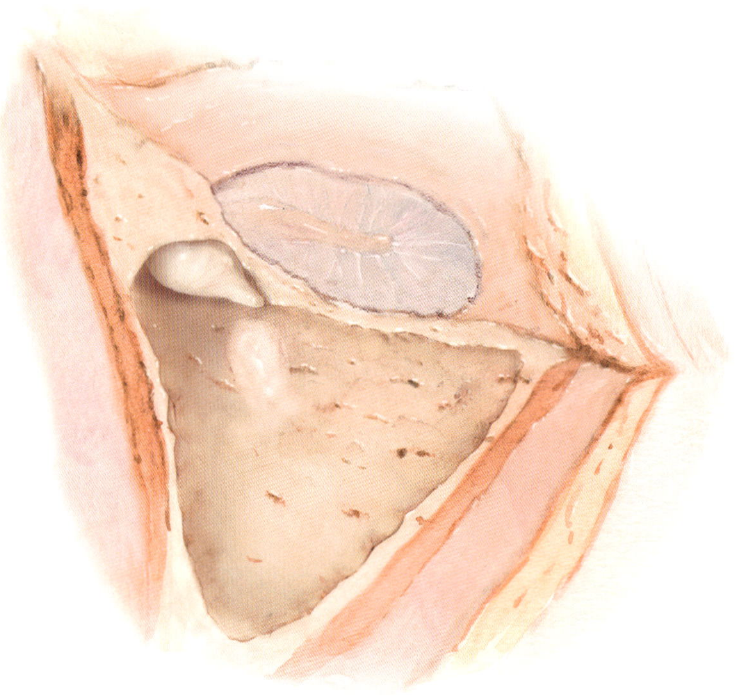

Fig. 6.15

Tip: Extensive tympanoatticotomy should be avoided and a transmastoid approach should be chosen instead. If tympanoatticotomy is performed with a drill, do not touch the ossicular chain. In anterior tympanotomy (pretubal cells), be careful of the facial nerve and geniculate ganglion.

Transmastoid Approaches

Mastoidectomy

A mastoidectomy is indicated as a first-line approach for other middle ear pathologies, such as acute mastoiditis and meningoencephalic herniation into the mastoid and middle ear, as well as cochlear implantation.

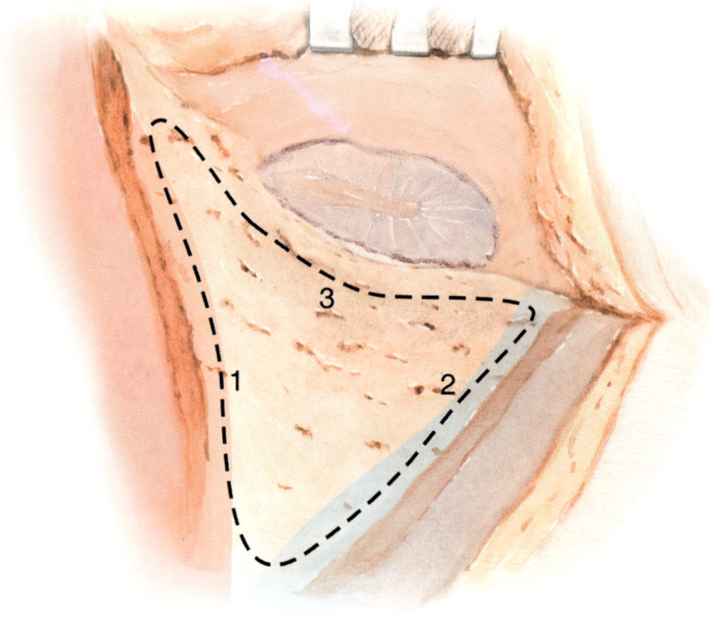

Fig. 6.16

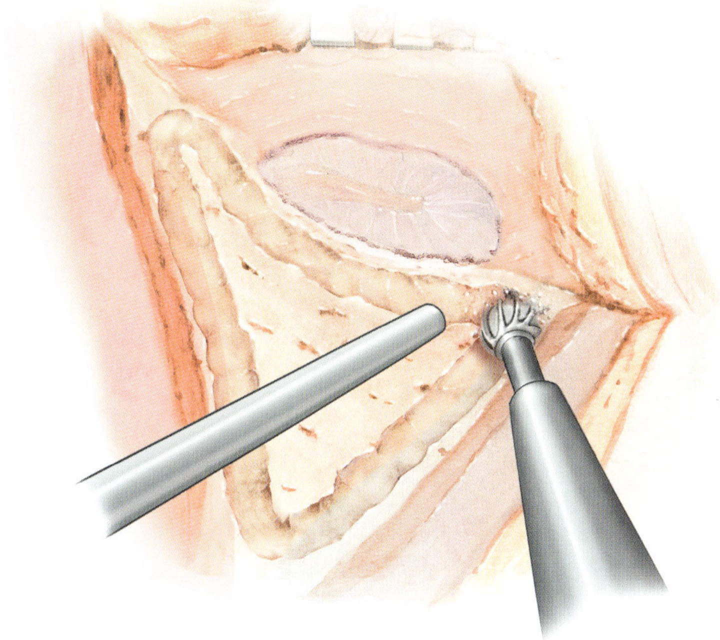

Fig. 6.17

Mastoid Landmark Identification

When the mastoid cortex is exposed, drilling with a large cutting burr should be started along the temporal line in an anteroposterior direction (1) to identify the middle fossa plate, followed by a posterior line to mark the sigmoid sinus (2). Finally, a third line is drilled just behind the posterior wall of the external auditory canal (3).

Fig. 6.16, Fig. 6.17

Tip: Structures can be easily identified. The temporal plate is pink with small vessels, and the sigmoid sinus is blue. Vision should be adjusted to be parallel to the posterior wall of the external auditory canal to estimate its thickness and axis. Burr movements should be parallel to important structures. It is better to enlarge the mastoidectomy rather than drill a deep narrow hole.

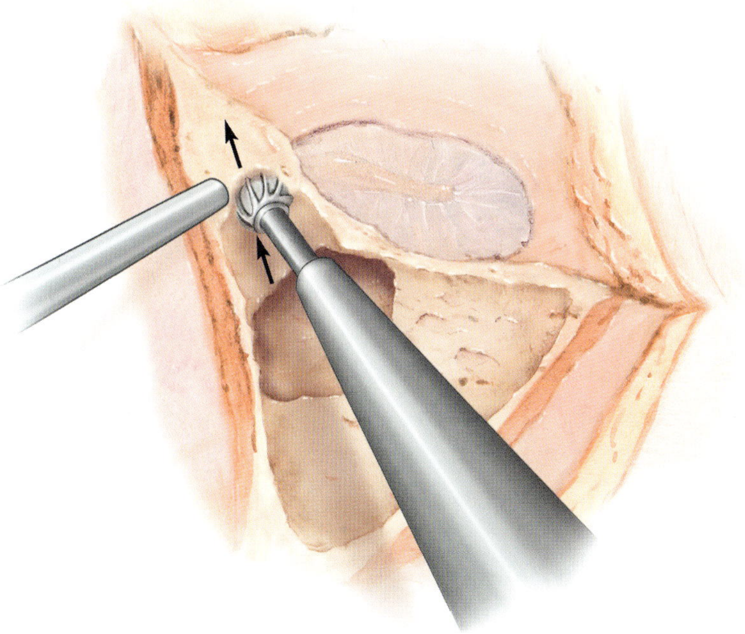

Fig. 6.18

Opening the Antrum

The next step is to find the antrum, which is situated between the posterosuperior angle of the external auditory canal and the anterior part of the temporal plate.

Fig. 6.18

Tip: The middle fossa plate may be situated low, hampering easy access to the antrum. The temporal plate and posterior bony wall should be thinned as much as possible. Significant temporal plate and external auditory canal defects should be fixed with bone pâté.

Opening of the Aditus

Once the antrum with its lateral semicircular canal has been identified, it should be carefully widened using a smaller cutting burr.

An anterior angle groove is drilled from medial to lateral to open the aditus.

Fig. 6.19

Tip: Care must be taken not to touch the short process of the incus, which can be visualized by rotating the patient's head forward. Use a diamond drill. If the incus needs to be removed for any reason, this should be done before attic drilling. Ossicular chain integrity should also be checked before drilling.

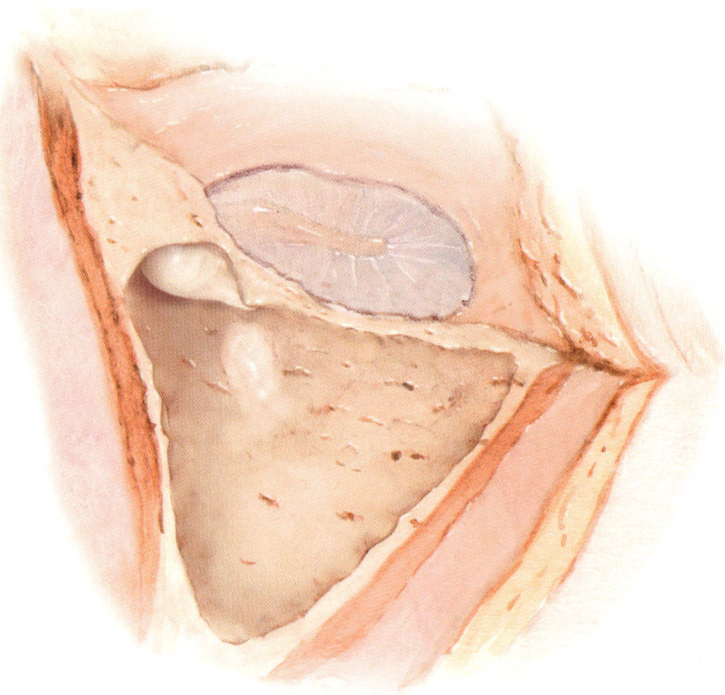

Fig. 6.19

Drilling the Mastoid Tip

Finally, any residual mastoid cells are drilled. The mastoid tip is opened, if required. To locate the facial nerve, the digastric ridge is identified first, as the facial nerve is situated just below its anterior level. The facial nerve is followed from inferior to superior.

Fig. 6.20

Tip: Be careful around the sinodural angle not to touch the superior petrosal sinus. The genu and mastoid segment of the facial nerve is always located under the incus short process axis. It can also be identified at the beginning of its third portion inferior to the lateral semicircular canal. Careful drilling should be performed with a diamond burr and abundant irrigation.

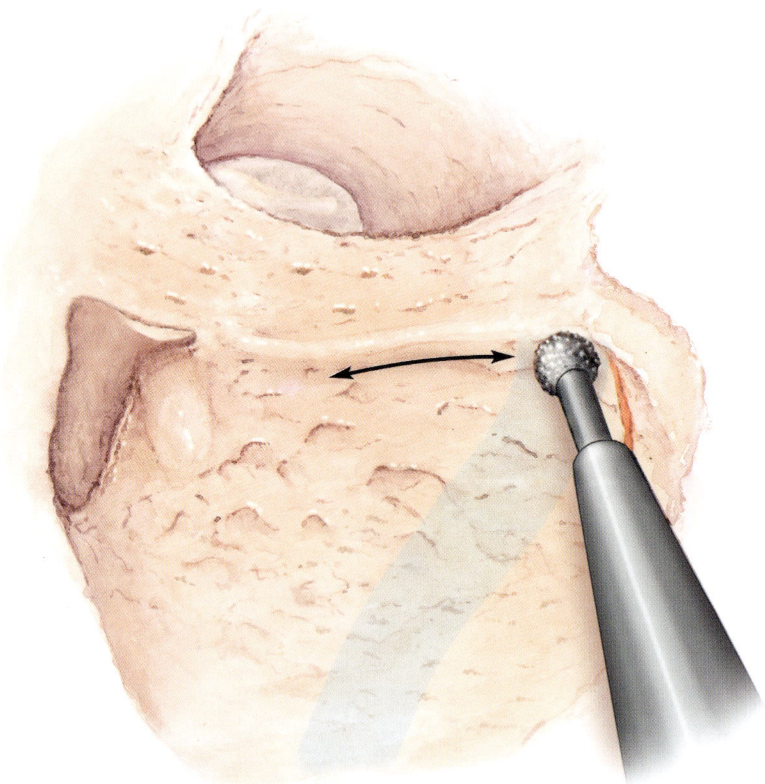

Fig. 6.20

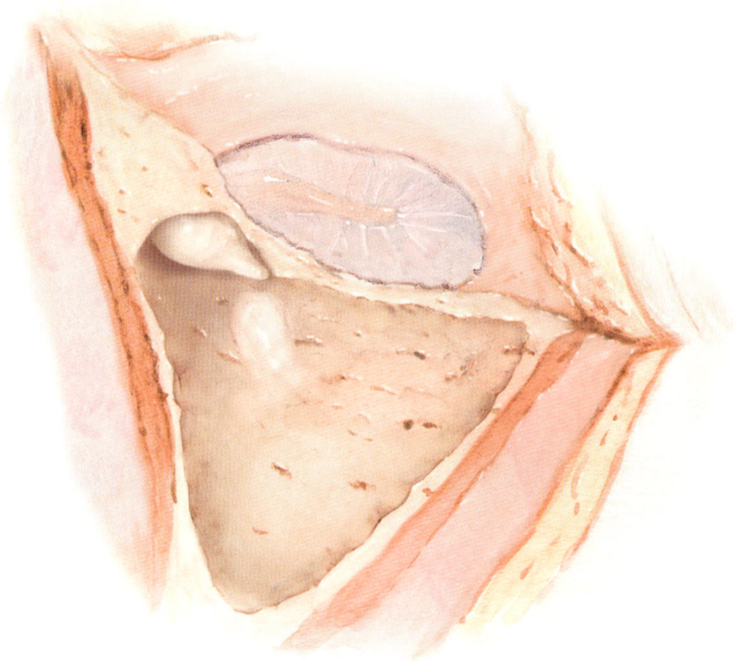

Fig. 6.21

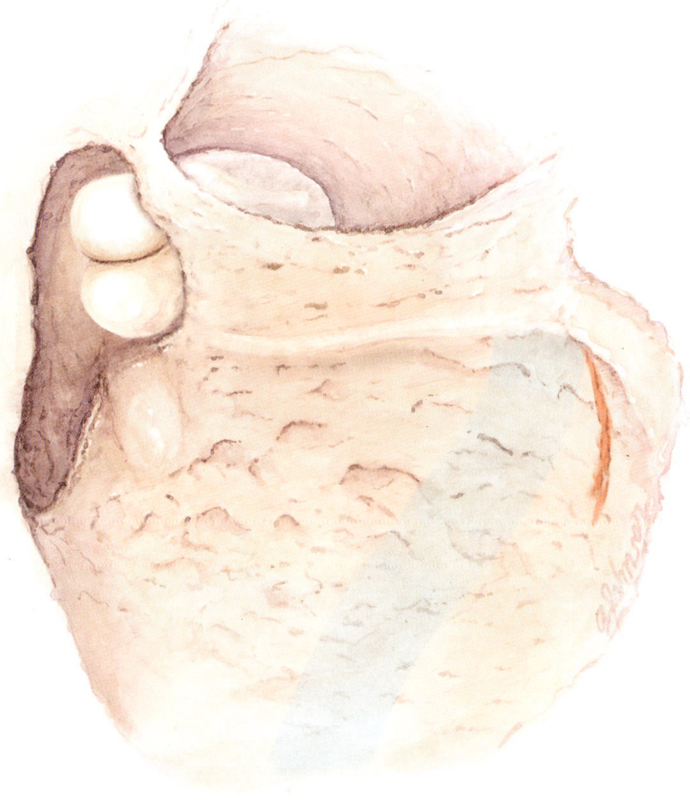

Fig. 6.22

Posterior Epitympanotomy

Opening the Anterior Angle

The anterior angle groove is continued from medial to lateral, keeping the superior bony canal wall intact, to expose the incus head.

Fig. 6.21

Exposure of Ossicle Heads

If the ossicular chain remains intact, drilling is performed using a diamond burr and the final bony overhang of the incus and malleus is removed using a curette or microhook.

When the posterior epitympanotomy is completed, the incus body and malleus head should be visible.

Fig. 6.22

Tip: Except in the case of incudomallear fixation, the incudostapedial joint is disarticulated before any transmastoid approach is initiated.

Exposure of Malleus Head
If the incudostapedial joint is discontinuous, the incus is removed and a cutting burr can be used to complete the posterior epitympanotomy.

Fig. 6.23

Exposure of Anterior Epitympanum
To reach the anterior epitympanum (pretubal cells), the incus and malleus head are first removed and the opening is then made using a diamond or cutting burr.

The cog is drilled out to reach the supratubal recess, paying particular attention to the facial nerve running along the inferior wall, and the geniculate ganglion located anteriorly.

Fig. 6.24

At the end, the whole attic, including the cog and anterior epitympanum, must be inspected.

Tip: Care must be taken not to injure the dura. Defects 0.5 cm in size should be repaired with bone pâté. If you need to take a risk, it is better to fenestrate the superior wall of the external auditory canal and reconstruct it with cartilage and bone pâté. Drill from medial to lateral so as not to touch the ossicular chain.

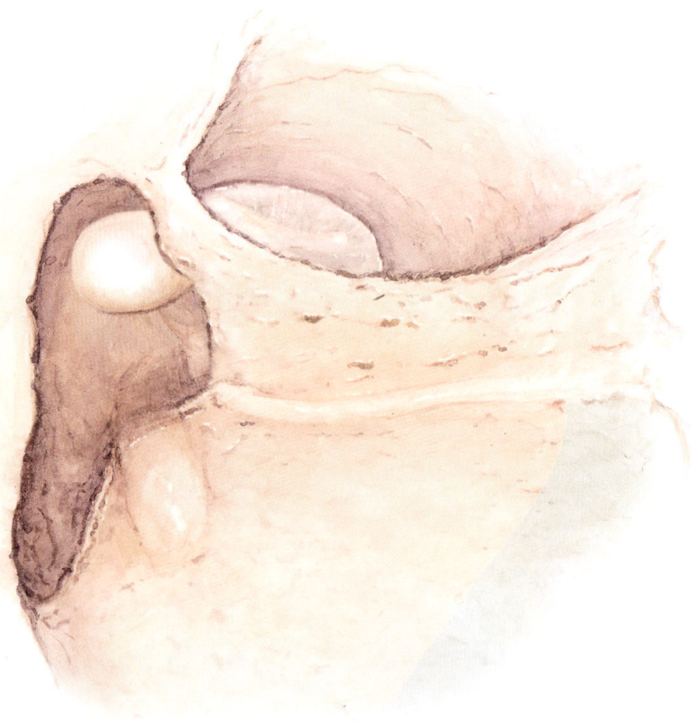

Fig. 6.23

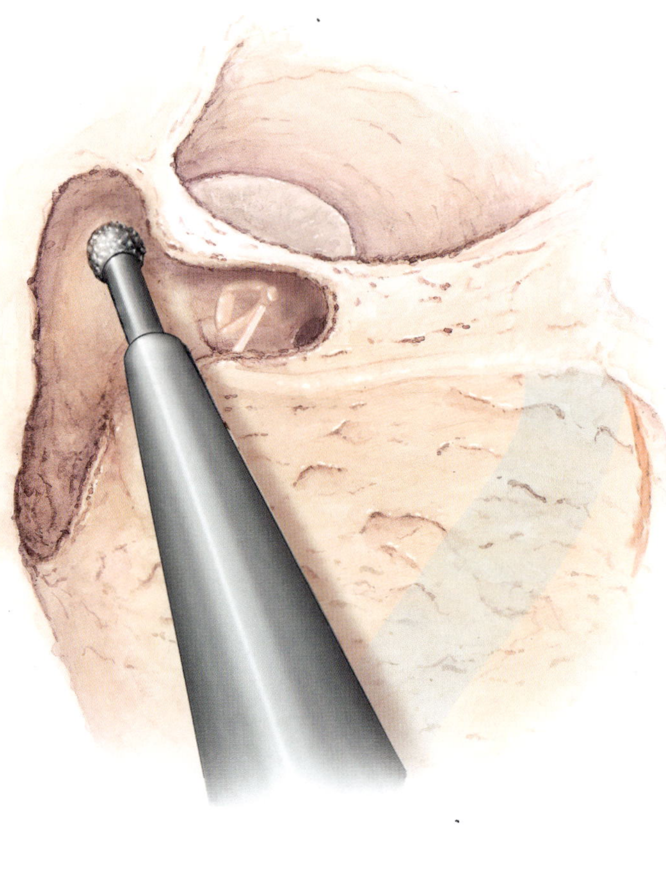

Fig. 6.24

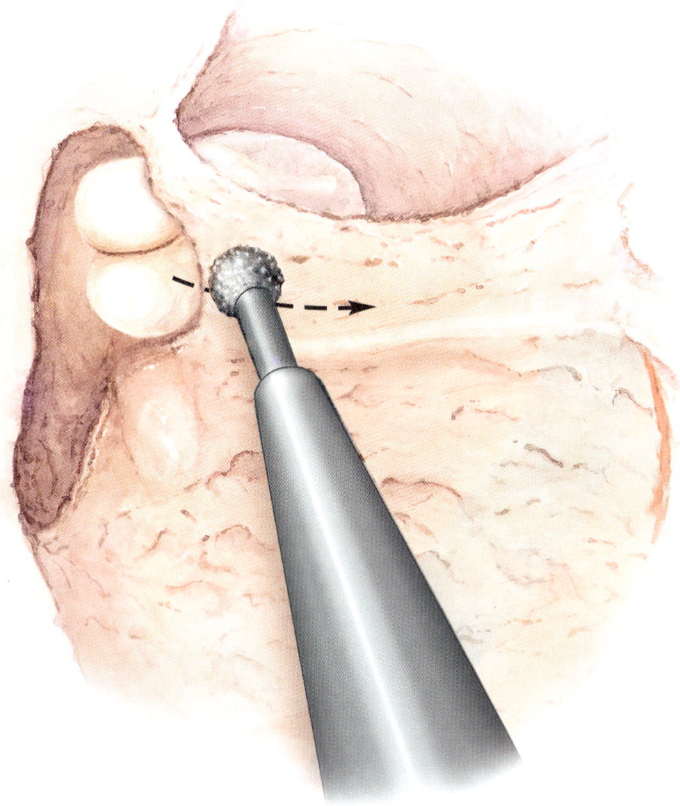

Fig. 6.25

Posterior Tympanotomy

Identification of Landmarks

After identification of the short process of the incus and the lateral semicircular canal, the posterior canal wall is thinned out using a large diamond burr.

With the same burr, a drilling groove is started in the short process axis continuity (or presumed axis, if removed). Facial recess cells are identified and drilled between the chorda tympani and the third portion of the facial nerve.

Fig. 6.25

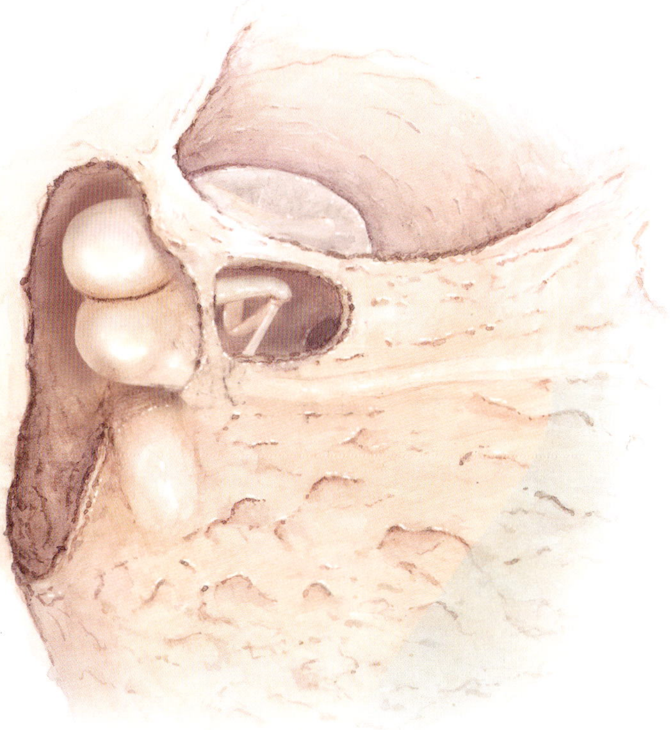

Fig. 6.26

Bony Buttress

If the incus can be preserved, a small bony buttress is kept intact between the incus short process and the posterior tympanotomy. To improve access to the oval window area, bone covering the facial nerve should be thinned using a diamond burr.

Fig. 6.26

Extended Posterior Tympanotomy
To check the round window or hypotympanic regions, the posterior tympanotomy should be extended inferiorly. The chorda tympani is drilled out and the posterior tympanotomy continued.
Fig. 6.27

Tip: Be careful of the facial nerve, which runs more laterally in its inferior portion.

Optimal Posterior Tympanotomy (Incus Absent)
If the incus is removed, the buttress is drilled out.
Fig. 6.28

Tip: If the facial recess cells are obliterated, positive identification of the facial nerve is reassuring and helps to locate the facial recess. Drilling parallel to the facial nerve using the largest diamond burr and abundant irrigation prevents injury to the facial nerve. Posteriorly, care is taken not to drill the posterior semicircular canal, and posterosuperiorly, the lateral semicircular canal. Another way of identifying the facial nerve in its mastoid portion is to drill the mastoid tip and locate the digastric ridge. The facial nerve runs just anteroinferiorly to this ridge.

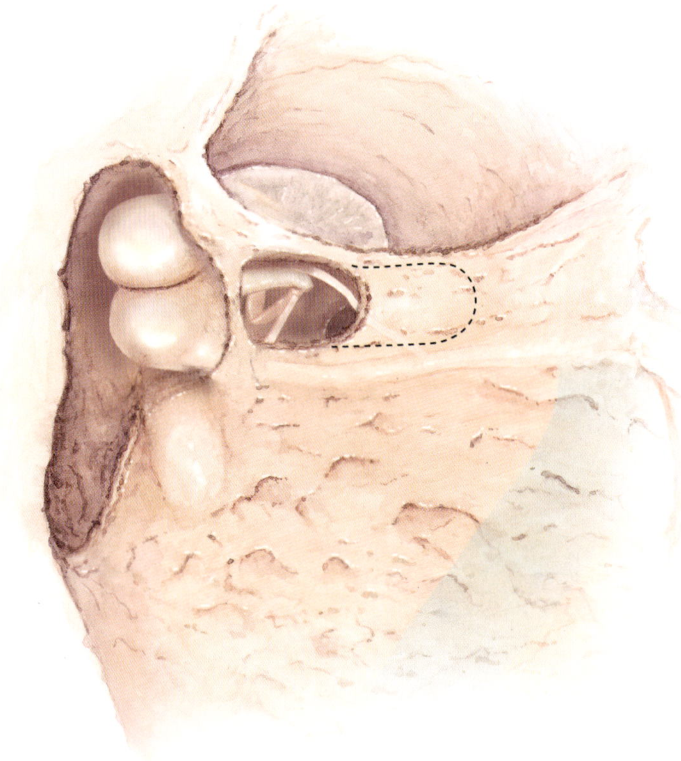

Fig. 6.27

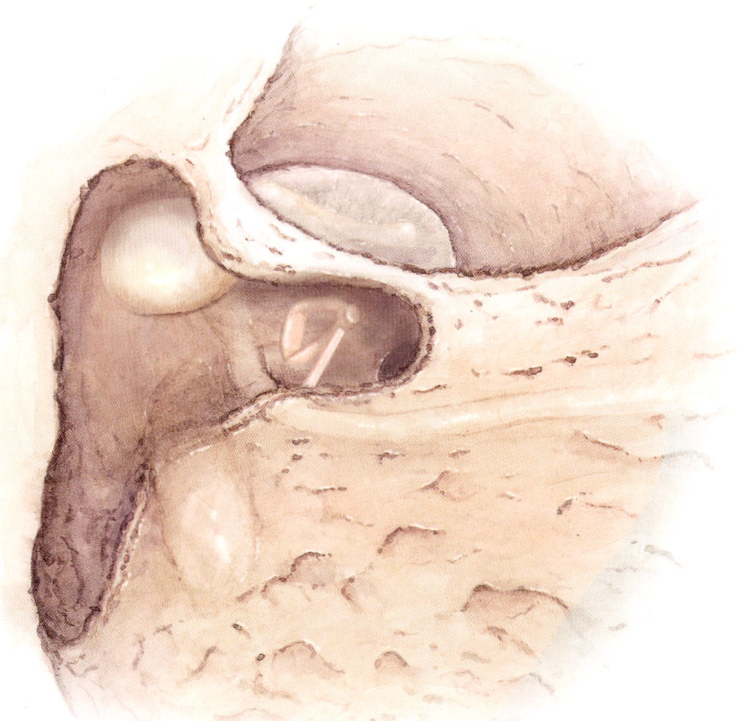

Fig. 6.28

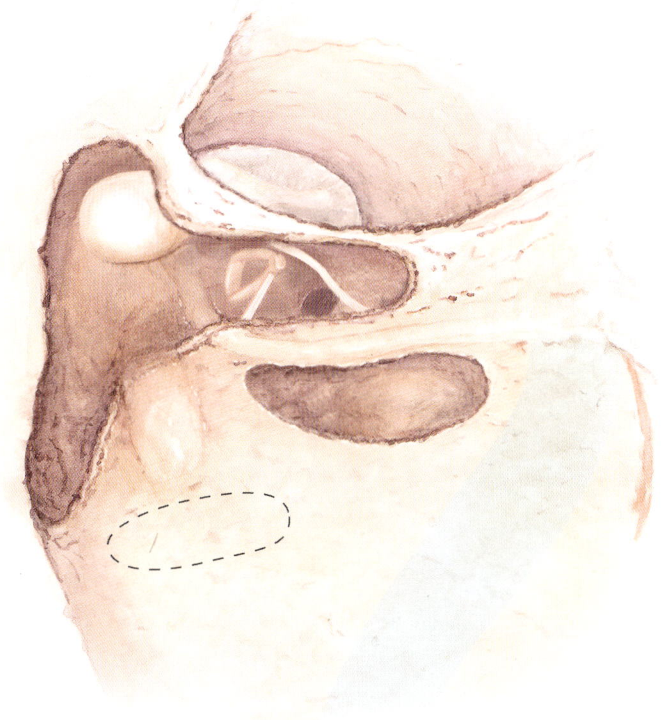

Fig. 6.29

Intersinofacial Approach

Drilling in Intersinofacial Approach

An intersinofacial approach should be reserved for specific pathologies involving the deep sinus tympani or extending under the third portion of the facial nerve. The entire third portion of the facial nerve is identified and the mastoid tip completely drilled. Sometimes the sigmoid sinus needs to be exposed and depressed to obtain a better view. Retrofacial cells are drilled out using a diamond burr until the sinus tympani is reached. **Fig. 6.29**

Tip: The patient's head should be rotated forward as far as possible. The cortical bone positioned superoposteriorly to the sigmoid sinus should be removed to improve the horizontal view. Care must be taken not to touch the inferior side of the facial nerve and the posterior semicircular canal (dotted line). The approach should be started in the mastoid tip region.

Middle Ear Pathology Management with a Canal-Wall-Up Technique

Middle ear pathologies are managed by a transmeatal approach and various transmastoid approaches. As much as possible should be done through the external auditory canal and epitympanic approach. Important structures like ossicles, round and oval windows, and the tympanic portion of the facial nerve should be identified and cleaned of pathological tissue, with incus removal if necessary. Once these fragile structures have been adequately managed, transmastoid drilling work can commence.

Cholesteatoma Management

Cholesteatoma Dissection

The best way to dissect a cholesteatoma is to follow the matrix and to keep it intact. Cholesteatoma debris can be removed prior to matrix dissection to facilitate identification of important and fragile structures. Using suction, the matrix is elevated and dissected using a lateral knife or dissector-elevator. **Fig. 6.30**

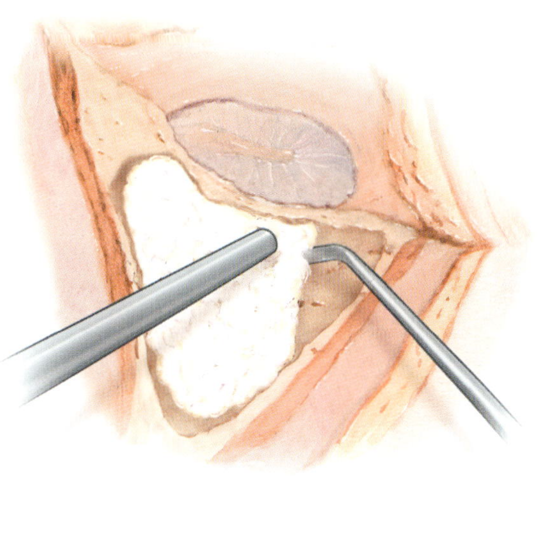

Fig. 6.30

Hypotympanic, Protympanic, and Mesotympanic Cholesteatoma

Hypotympanic cholesteatomas sometimes extend between the carotid artery and the jugular bulb, and inferior tympanotomy may be required (see Posterior Epitympanotomy, p. 114). If the inferior tympanotomy is insufficient, a definitive (with or without rehabilitation) canal-wall-down (CWD) technique should be performed (see Canal-Wall-Down Rehabilitation, p. 132).

The jugular bulb is extremely fragile, therefore dissection or drilling (with a diamond burr) should be performed very carefully.

Tip: In cases where there is jugular bulb damage and bleeding, Surgicel (Johnson & Johnson, Cincinnati, Ohio, USA) is packed into the hypotympanic region.

Mesotympanic cholesteatomas include those involving the oval and round windows. These structures are approached through the meatus with or without posterior tympanoatticotomy.

Stapes Dissection

A cholesteatoma of the stapes superstructure is carefully dissected with a needle and small-diameter suction, respecting the long axis of the stapes.

Fig. 6.31

Stapedial Arch Dissection

When the matrix is underneath the stapes arch, a small, soaked cotton ball is pushed through the arch using a needle or microhook.

Fig. 6.32

If any residual matrix is suspected, the superstructure should be removed by laser or microscissors (see Removal of the Stapes Superstructure, p. 77).

When the stapedial tendon, chorda tympani, or pyramidal eminence are covered with cholesteatomas, the same strategy should be applied: careful cleaning or removal.

When the superstructure is absent and the footplate shows extensive cholesteatoma involvement, the dissection is performed from posterior to anterior using a needle or dissector-elevator.

Tip: If an opened vestibule is suspected, the matrix should be left on the footplate and second-stage surgery planned within the year.

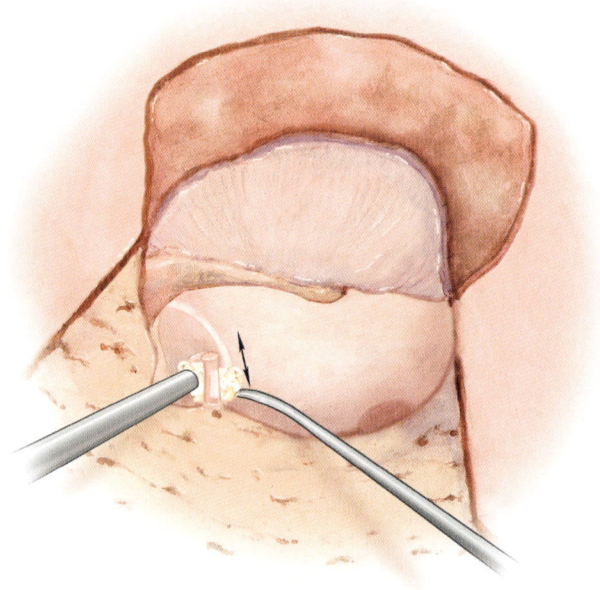

Fig. 6.31

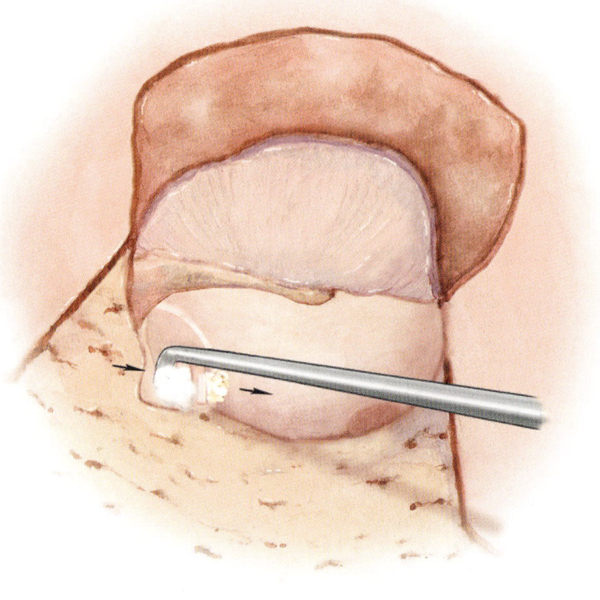

Fig. 6.32

Facial Nerve Dissection

When the facial nerve is covered with the matrix, careful dissection is performed using a small-diameter suction, and a dissector-elevator to push through a soaked cotton ball. The long axis of the nerve is respected at all times.

Fig. 6.33

Malleus Removal

To access the protympanic area, any residual manubrium should be removed after tendon section of the tensor tympani muscle.

Fig. 6.34

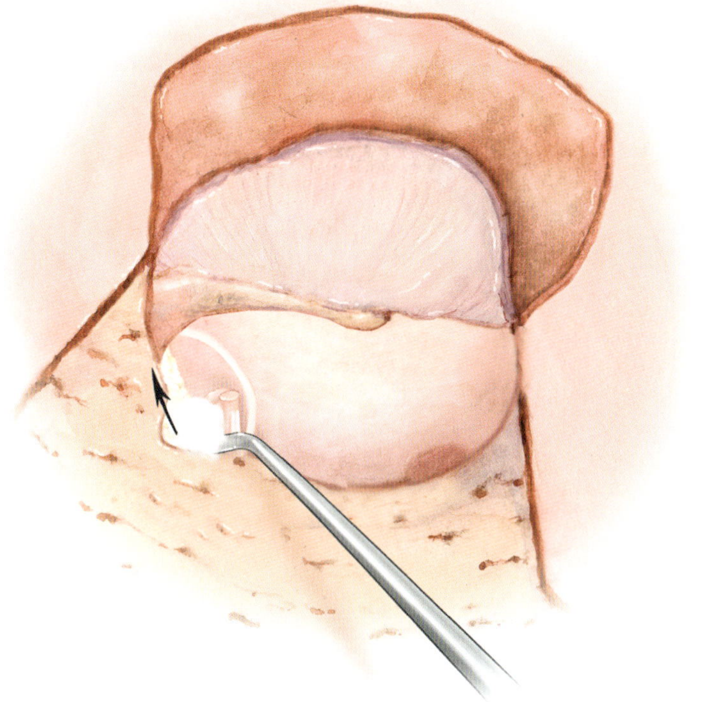

Fig. 6.33

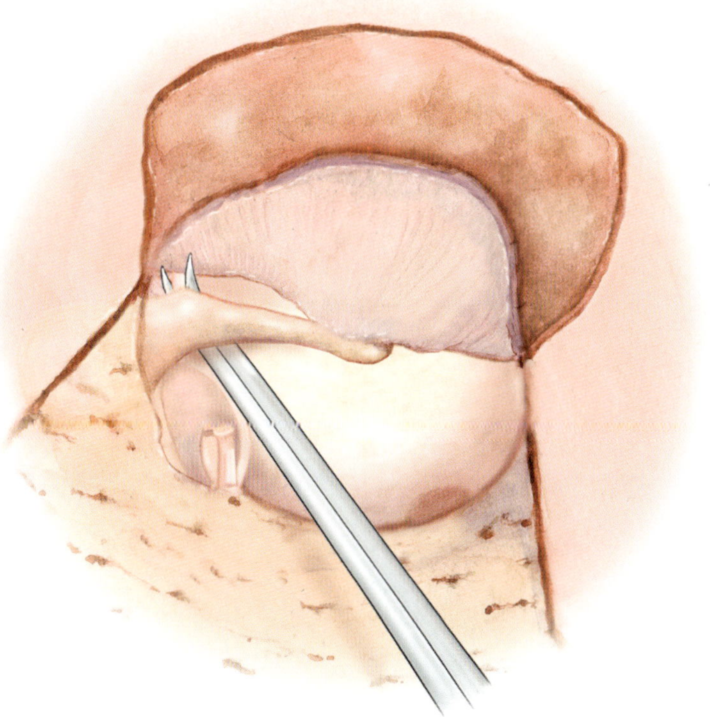

Fig. 6.34

Retrotympanic Cholesteatoma

With uncontrolled cholesteatoma extension to the facial recess and sinus tympani, dissection requires a combined approach (transmeatal and posterior tympanotomy).

Sinus Tympani Dissection

A soaked cotton ball is pushed into the sinus tympani using a dissector-elevator. If the sinus tympani is extremely deep, an intersinofacial approach might be required (see Intersinofacial Approach, p. 121).

Fig. 6.35

Tip: Otoendoscopes or Zini mirrors can be used to confirm cholesteatoma removal.

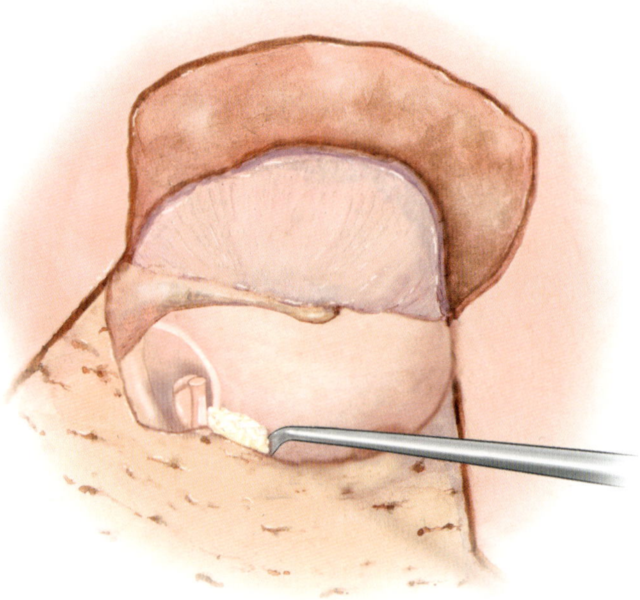

Fig. 6.35

Attic Cholesteatoma

Extended cholesteatomas of the attic regions are managed by a combined approach: transmeatal and posterior epitympanotomy with or without posterior tympanoatticotomy.

Incus and Malleus Head Removal

When the incus is surrounded by cholesteatomas, it should be removed and cannot be use for incus interposition (see Removal of the Incus, p. 90).

When the malleus head shows matrix involvement, the head is removed after the neck, cutting through the meatus with a malleus nipper.

Fig. 6.36

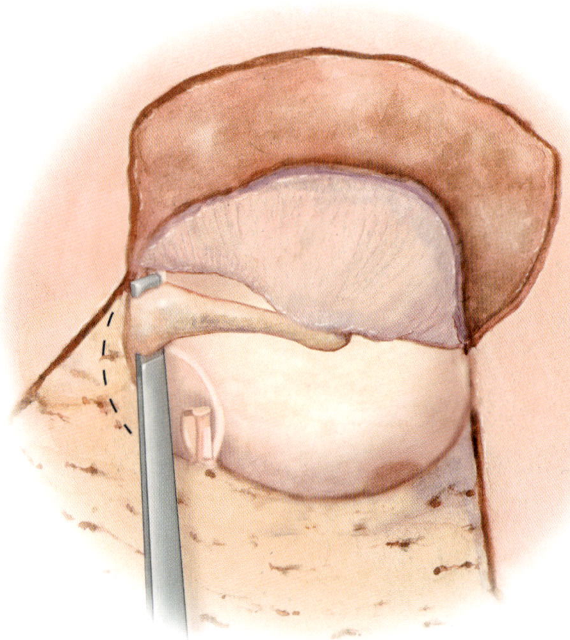

Fig. 6.36

Attical Dissection
The matrix is slowly elevated using suction and a dissector-elevator with or without a soaked cotton ball.

Fig. 6.37

Dissection of the Anterior Attic
If the cholesteatoma extends to the anterior epitympanum, the residual cog is drilled away to reach the supratubal recess, taking particular care around the facial nerve running along the bottom wall.

Fig. 6.38

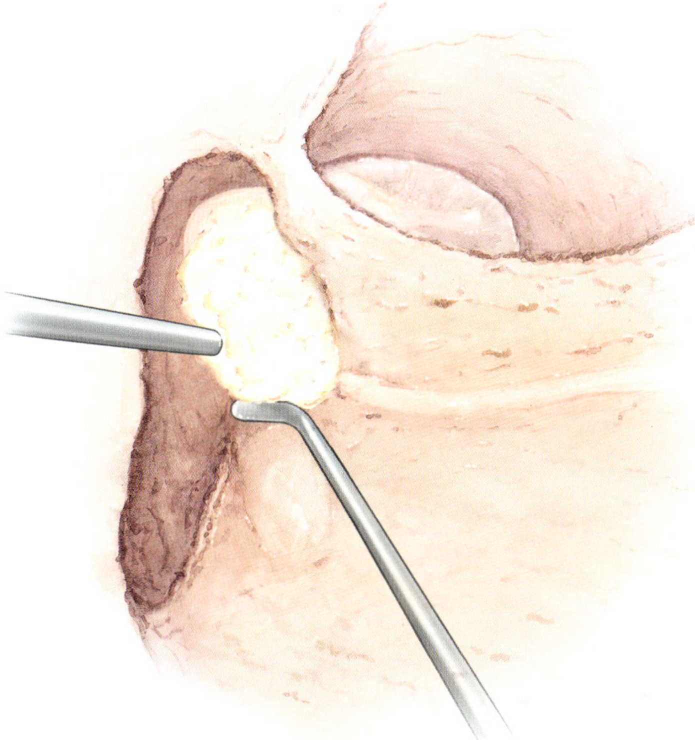

Fig. 6.37

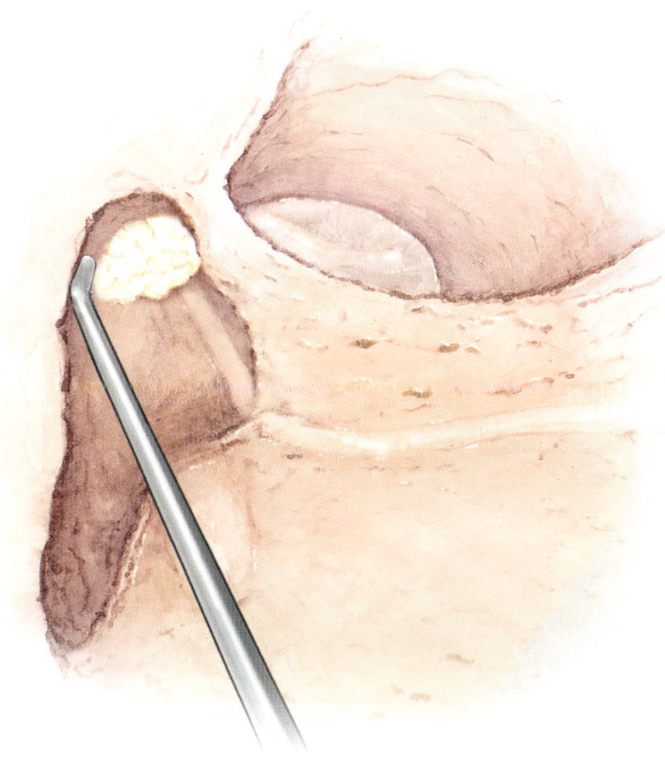

Fig. 6.38

Supratubal Recess Dissection
This area is cleaned using a combined approach (transmeatal and posterior epitympanotomy).
Fig. 6.39

Tip: Care should be taken around the geniculate ganglion located anterior to the supratubal recess. Cells should be drilled out until flat and healthy bone is reached using a diamond burr. Do not forget to drill and clean the perilabyrinthine cells.

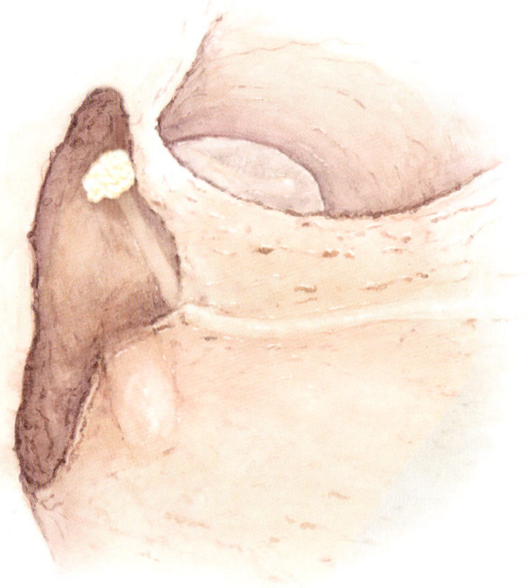

Fig. 6.39

Cholesteatoma Extension to the Mastoid and Antrum

Mastoid and antral cholesteatomas require mastoidectomy (see Mastoidectomy, p. 114).

In the mastoid, cells may be infiltrated by cholesteatoma. In such cases, the cells should be drilled with a diamond burr until flat and healthy bone is reached.

In antral cholesteatoma, there is a risk of labyrinthine fistula. Careful dissection is required around the lateral semicircular canal and, if a fistula is suspected, it is managed at the end of the cholesteatoma dissection.

Tip: Do not drill into the cholesteatoma, as it causes extensive epidermic debris. Dissect first and drill after.

Dissection of Canal Fistula
With fistulas, a small temporalis fascia or perichondrium graft is prepared behind the fistula. The matrix is slowly pushed out using a round knife without using suction around the fistula.
Fig. 6.40

Tip: A cotton ball or Merocel can facilitate dissection.

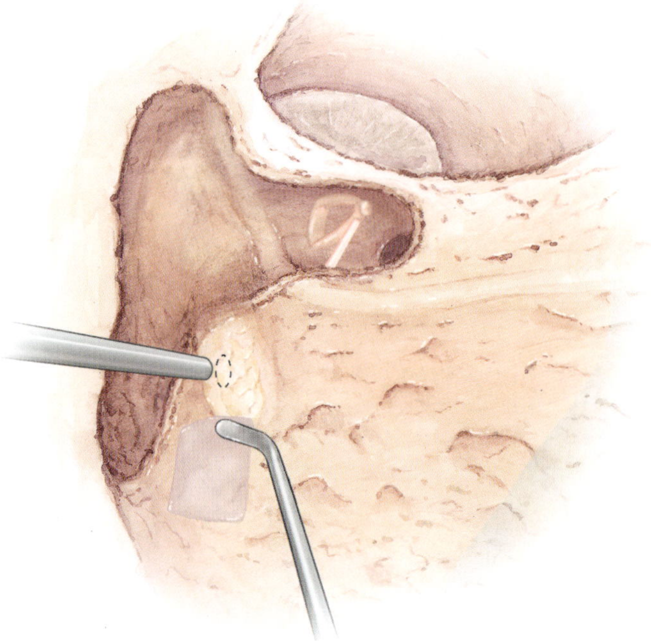

Fig. 6.40

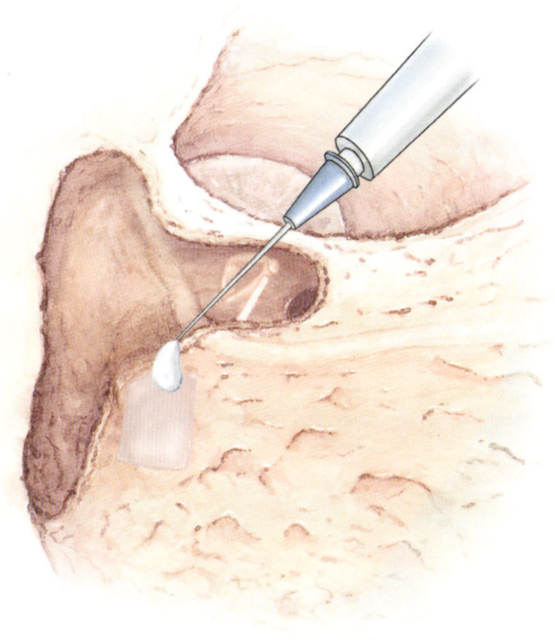

Fig. 6.41

Fistula Graft Placement

The graft is placed on the fistula and fixed with fibrin glue. If matrix adhesions are too extensive, the matrix is trimmed as much as possible around the fistula and second-stage surgery is planned within the year.

Fig. 6.41

Tip: It is easier and safer to remove a cholesteatoma pearl during second-stage surgery.

Tip: Even if the fistula is very large, a CWD procedure is avoided as far as possible to prevent vertigo caused by wind and cavity cleaning.

Revision and Second-Stage Surgery

Second-stage surgery is considered in the case of large and aggressive cholesteatomas, uncontrolled stapes cholesteatomas, infected cholesteatomas, large bony defects, mucosal inflammation, and poor middle ear ventilation.

Revision surgery is performed in the case of functional failure, residual cholesteatoma suspected on follow-up CT scan or MRI, and recurrent cholesteatomas.

The approach depends on where the disease is located. For cholesteatomas situated in the epitympanum, antrum, and mastoid, a retroauricular approach is applied. If the cholesteatoma is located in the tympanic cavity, a transcanal approach is preferred, but the retroauricular approach should remain an alternative option if the transcanal approach does not result in satisfactory management.

Tip: Otoendoscopes may be useful in this type of surgery.

Canal-Wall-Down Technique

CWD technique is used in only 3 % of our cholesteatoma procedures. Our indications for CWD are:

- Large defects of the external auditory bony canal wall with mastoid erosion
- Significant recurrence of cholesteatomas after CWU
- Very large labyrinthine fistulas
- Extensive cholesteatomas in patients who are high-risk candidates for anesthesia or likely to be unreliable for follow-up

Removal of the Canal bony Wall

When the tympanomeatal flap has been elevated, the incus and malleus heads have been removed, and a mastoidectomy and an atticoantrotomy have been performed, the external auditory canal posterior wall is removed using a cutting burr with a parallel movement to the facial nerve from lateral to medial.

Fig. 6.42

Facial Ridge Drilling

When the facial ridge is approached, a diamond burr follows the course of the facial nerve. The ridge should be thinned as much as possible without exposing the nerve.

Fig. 6.43

Tip: It is important to saucerize the cavity by removing bony overhangs and small cells using a large diamond burr. The cavity should be flat and round.
All the bone covering the sigmoid sinus and fossa dura should be very thin.
Preserving the malleus handle helps to reconstruct a better columellar effect, which improves functional results. Do not forget the mastoid tip cells, and be careful of the facial nerve which runs just anterior to the digastric ridge.

Tympanic Membrane Reconstruction

The type of tympanic membrane reconstruction undertaken depends on eustachian tube function.

If it is functional, a pseudo middle ear cavity is reconstructed using a large tragal perichondrium–cartilage graft. The graft is positioned underlying the residual tympanic membrane or

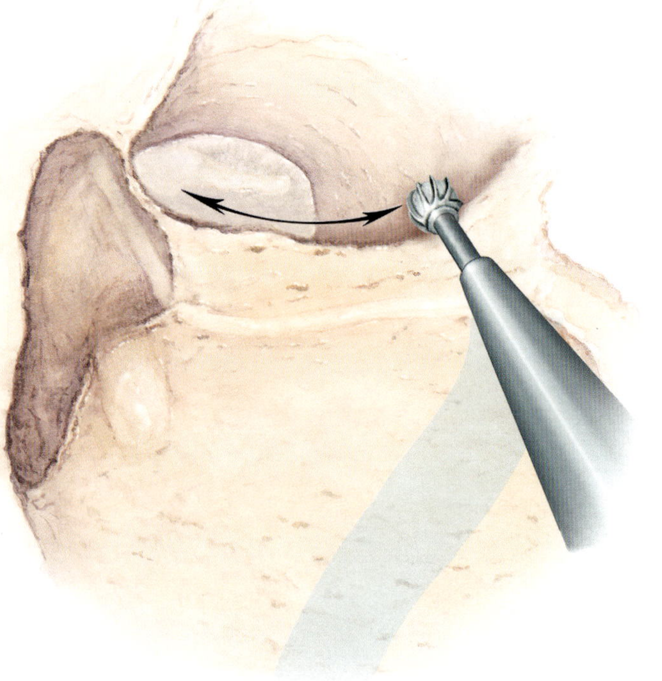

Fig. 6.42

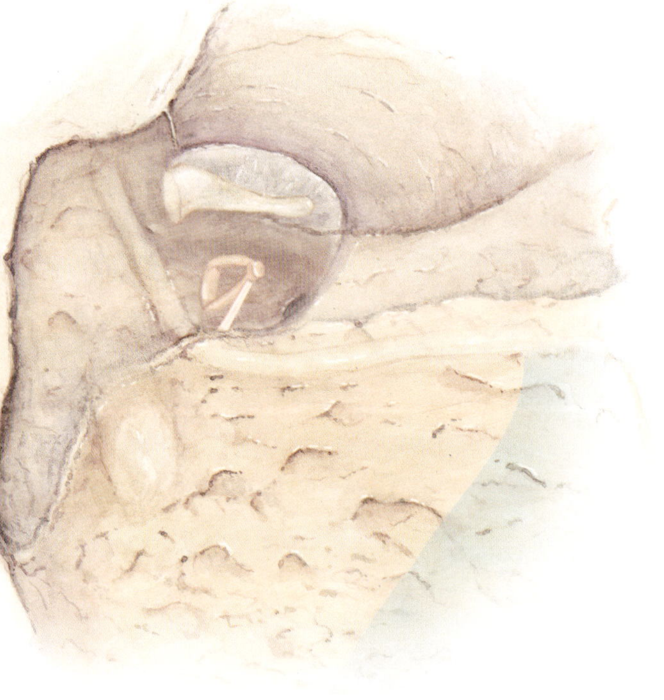

Fig. 6.43

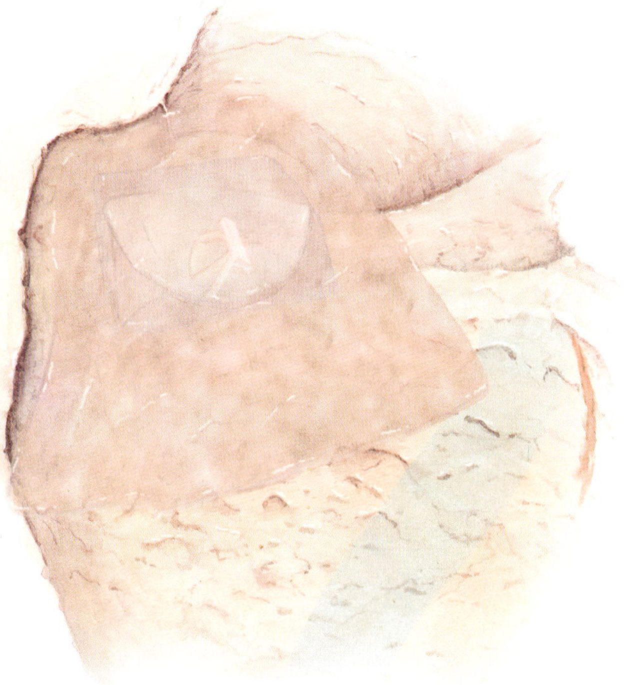

Fig. 6.44

overlying the sulcus. The cartilage–perichondrium covers the middle ear cavity, and the perichondrium, the facial ridge and attic. With an intact stapes superstructure, the cartilage is positioned on the stapes capitulum. Without a superstructure, a small cartilage piece can be placed on the footplate to guarantee a columellar effect between the footplate and tragal cartilage. An ossiculoplasty can also be performed with a prosthesis.

If the eustachian tube is not functional, only temporalis fascia is used to reconstruct the pseudo middle ear cavity. No ossiculoplasty is performed.

Tip: The prosthesis used will be shorter because it only extends to the facial ridge.

Finally, temporalis fascia is placed on the uncovered attic area and the largest surface of the mastoid.

Fig. 6.44

Tip: A large temporalis fascia graft facilitates epithelialization.

Large Mastoid Cavity Obliteration

A prominent, well-pneumatized mastoid tip and/or large cavity should be partially obliterated. A posteroinferior soft tissue flap is used for the mastoid tip and a posterosuperior flap for the retrofacial and retrolabyrinthine cells. A free temporal muscle flap can be considered and placed in the posterior part of the mastoidectomy to reduce its size.

Meatoplasty

To facilitate cavity ventilation and office cleaning of your cavity, a meatoplasty should always be performed. We perform meatoplasty at the end of the surgical procedure before closure.

Lateral Incisions

Using a nasal speculum, two lateral incisions are made in the meatus (skin, cartilage, and connective tissue) with a no. 11 scalpel.
Fig. 6.45

Skin Dissection

By a transcanal approach, the skin tissue is dissected using pointed curved scissors to reach the conchal cartilage. The meatal skin is elevated from the cartilage.
Fig. 6.46

Cartilage Removal

A piece of conchal cartilage shaped like a nail is removed. Using the retroauricular approach, the meatal skin flap is folded posteriorly and sutured to the connective tissue using 3/0 Vicryl.
Fig. 6.47

Packing and Closure

Soaked Spongostan is packed into the whole cavity. The musculoperiosteal and retroauricular flaps are sutured. A Merocel Schindler ear pack is used to help meatoplasty calibration.

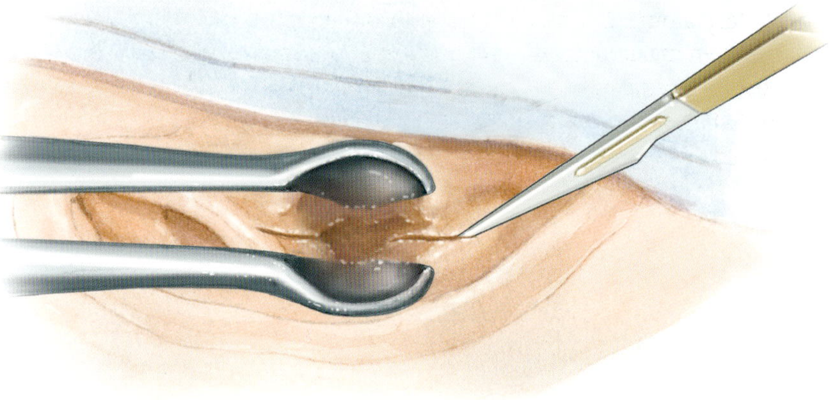

Fig. 6.45

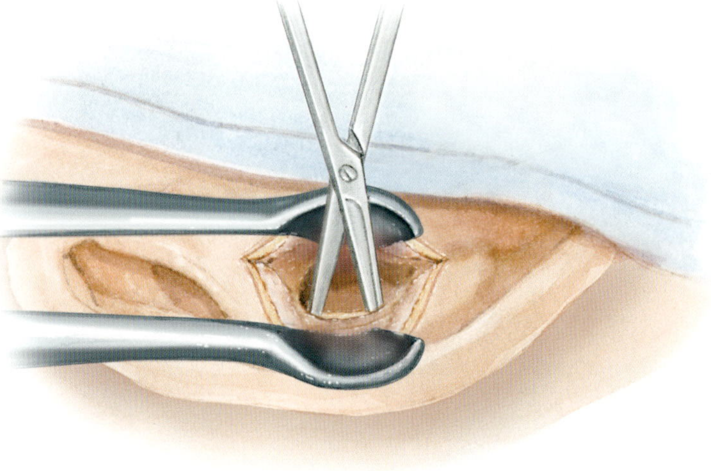

Fig. 6.46

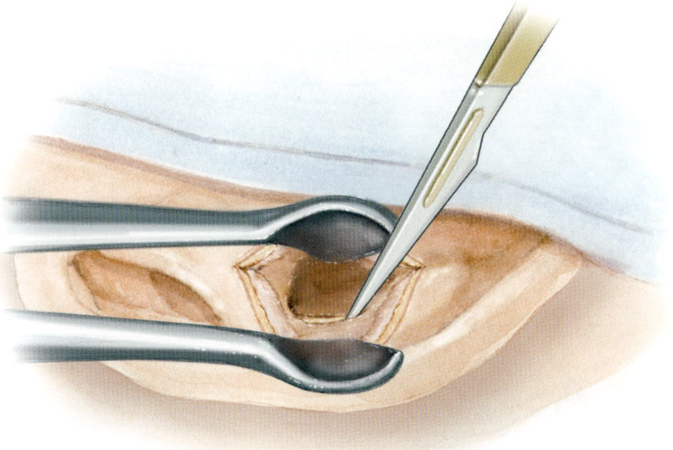

Fig. 6.47

Paratympanic Cavity Obliteration Technique

This technique, first described by Mercke (1987), may be considered in cases of multiple recurrence of or extended epitympanic cholesteatoma. Unlike the CWD technique, it preserves the physiological appearance of the external auditory canal, but there is a risk of enclosed residual cholesteatoma. Good-quality imaging follow-up is required.

When mastoidectomy and posterior epitympanotomy with or without posterior tympanotomy are completed, and there are no bony overhangs, just a flat, round cavity without any mucosal remnants, obliteration is initiated.

Paratympanic Cavity Isolation

Through the meatus, a temporalis fascia or perichondrial graft is placed between the facial ridge (tympanic segment and possibly mastoid segment) and tympanic membrane frame.

Fig. 6.48

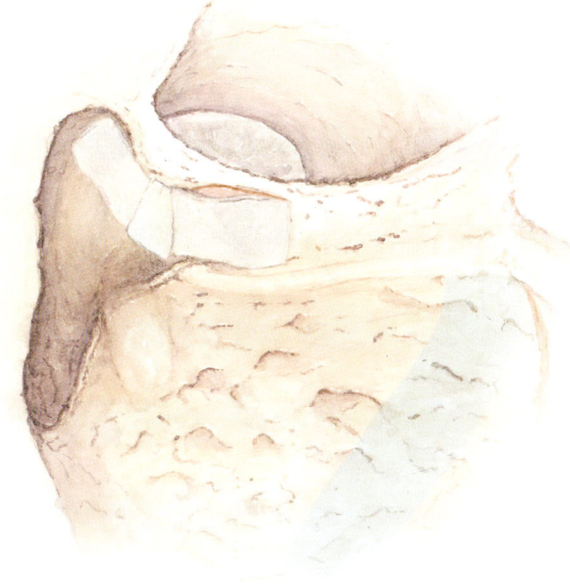

Fig. 6.48

Paratympanic and Mastoid Cavity Filling

Through the mastoidectomy, cartilage chips (autografts or allografts) are positioned behind the temporalis fascia or perichondrial graft. Fibrin glue is added. Bone pâté is prepared with bone dust from the patient or a tissue bank. Hydroxyapatite cement or a fascia later allograft can also be used.

The whole epitympanic area and mastoid is filled with one of these preparations.

Fig. 6.49

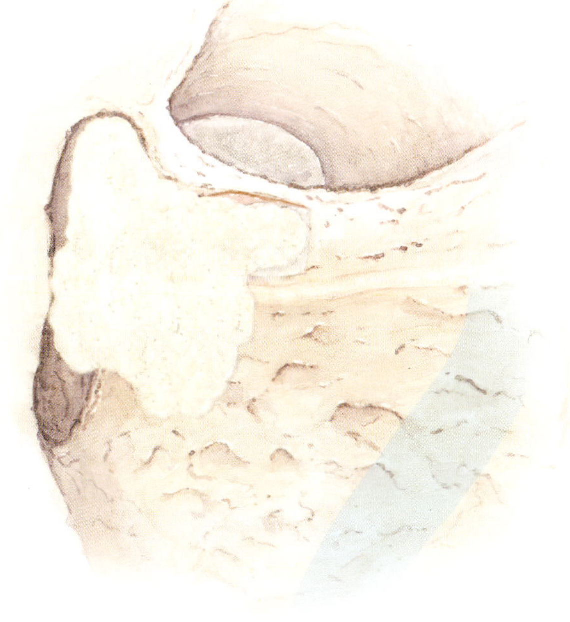

Fig. 6.49

Tip: Do not leave any mucosal or epidermic remnants in the cavity. If in doubt, employ the CWD technique.

Canal-Wall-Down Rehabilitation

External Auditory Canal Reconstruction

The external auditory bony canal wall is first reconstructed with a fascia lata allograft or Tutopatch from the facial ridge to the mastoid surface.

The rest of the obliteration procedure is the same as for paratympanic space obliteration.
Fig. 6.50

Tip: If a partial resection of the meatal bony wall is required for removal of pathological matter, the bony defect can be reconstructed with fascia lata or a Tutopatch.

The same principle is applied as for paratympanic space obliteration.

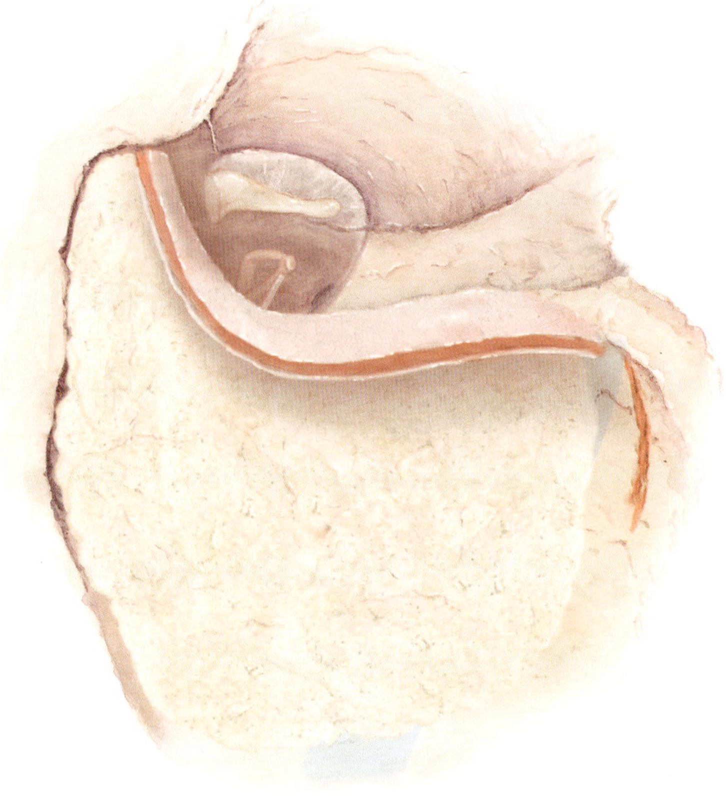

Fig. 6.50

Middle Ear Obliteration Technique

Middle ear obliteration involves filling the middle ear cavity with fat, blind sac closure of the external auditory canal, and eustachian tube closure with bone wax.

Indications for middle ear obliteration are:

- Open cavity with chronic inflammation and nonfunctional hearing
- Recurrent meningitis or CSF leakage from a temporal bone fracture
- Inoperable meningoencephalocele
- Cochlear implantation and chronic otitis media with risk of chronic inflammation

Middle Ear Cavity Preparation

A CWD is performed. The tympanic membrane, malleus, and incus are removed. The mastoid and middle ear cavity must be free of mucosa, and the residual part of the external auditory canal free of epithelium.

The proximal eustachian tube area is cleaned of its mucosa and plugged with bone wax.

Fig. 6.51

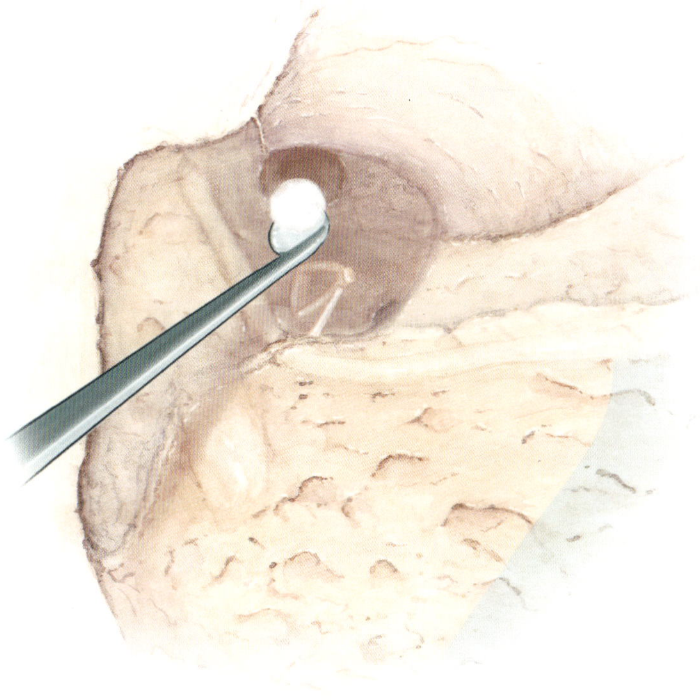

Fig. 6.51

Blind Sac Closure

Blind sac closure of the meatus is performed after transection of the meatal skin and cartilage proximally and elevation of the skin from the cartilage by several millimeters. Using a retroauricular approach the meatal skin is sutured with inside-out stitches using Vicryl.

The Vicryl is passed through the meatus and a knot is made on the outside. Before closure, the cavity is filled with abdominal fat and the musculoperiosteal flap is replaced to cover the meatal closure. The skin is closed in two layers.

Fig. 6.52

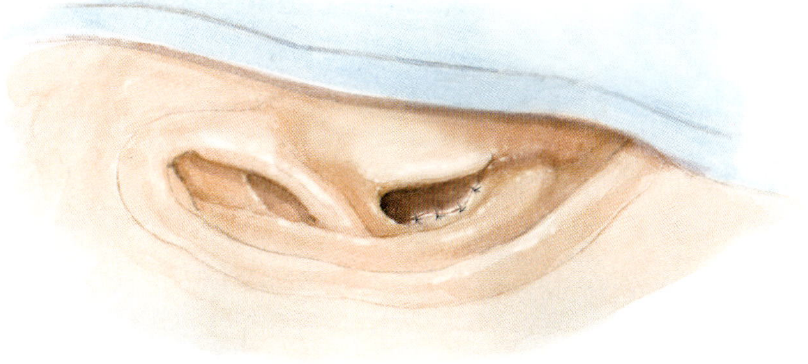

Fig. 6.52

7

Dressing and Postoperative Care

7__Dressing and Postoperative Care

For retroauricular incisions, a piece of gauze is cut and placed behind the auricle, while another piece covers the auricle. A circular Velpeau bandage holds the gauzes in place.

Except for noninfected type I tympanoplasty and stapes surgery, patients receive oral antibiotics for 1 week. The dressing is removed 24 hours after surgery and the Merocel Schindler ear pack just prior to discharge. Ciprofloxacin drops are applied twice a day until the Spongostan is completely removed (from 2 weeks postoperatively for stapes surgery to 4 weeks postoperatively for tympanoplasty with a large healing surface). When Epifilm is used, it remains in place until spontaneously rejected. Stitches, Steri-Strips, or cutaneous glue are removed after 1 week. Sometimes, the topical treatment is adjusted according to the healing process (corticosteroids or silver nitrate).

Index

Page numbers in *italics* refer to illustrations